Mother's Helpmates

Guide to Child Care- Nannies and Companions

We Answer Questions on Screening, Taxes, Salaries and More

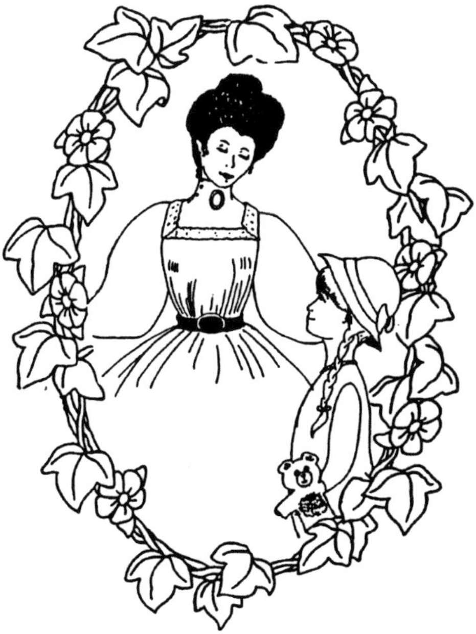

Cora Hilton Thomas

Book illustrations by: Valerie Hogan
Editorial Consultant: Jeff Corydon III

Library of Congress Catalog Number: 94-76905
ISBN 0-9642214-0-3

Printed in the United States of America
by Eric Statham, Pro Copy Inc.
5209 Fowler Ave., Tampa, FL 33617

Cover printed by Chuck McManus
Carrollwood Copy Center and Printing Inc.
10428 North Dale Mabry Hwy.
Tampa, FL 33618

God bless all the children big and small for on this earth they have no choice, they have no voice.

God bless all the children for the world they see will never be what it seems to be.

Light their path when the darkness surrounds them. Give them love, let it glow, all around them.

God bless all the children shield them from all harm, keep them safe, keep them warm.

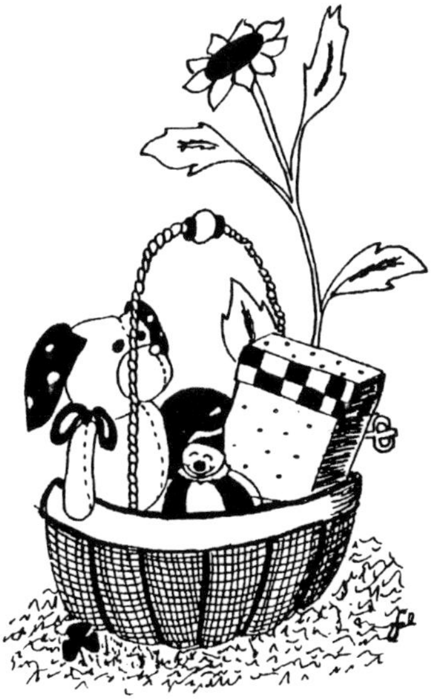

Dedication

This book is dedicated to my children Stephen, Alecia, and Ryan and husband, Scott, for all their patience and support while I wrote it, and to the loving memory of my mother, the best mother of all Cora Mae Chalk Hilton (1930-1976) taught me the importance of a mother's loving guidance in a child's life.

Acknowledgements

I am grateful for all the help, support and information I have received from many clients and from the following other sources in writing this book: Jeff Corydon III; Valerie Hogan for her art; The Tampa/ Hillsborough county library system for assisting with research; and The Criminal Justice Department in Washington D.C. and various state law enforcement agencies for their contributions.

Cora Hilton Thomas

TABLE OF CONTENTS

Table of Contents cont'd

INTRODUCTION

Mother's Helpmates aims to provide loving parents all the information they need to find safe, high-quality child care. Every child deserves the best and most professional care that a mother and father can afford, whether in a day care center or at home. This book answers the questions most parents have when considering child care. It provides, in one convenient guide, all the information you need to hire in-home help or arrange day care without the cost of an agency. If you are wondering what kind of care is best for your child or what the cost of a nanny is, it will clear up any questions you have. It gives a detailed outline of procedures a nanny placement agency uses when screening household help for families, information gathered through years of research and experience in placing help with families having both normal and special needs. Even if you are already using an agency, this guide will explain exactly what is involved in hiring household help so you know what you should be getting. The benefits of having a nanny vs. taking your child to a day care center are outlined, to help you and your family make the choice. What you will read in these pages is the precious information I needed and acquired as a mother, then used to found Mother's Helpmates. With today's rampant fears of child abuse making the search for quality child care more daunting than ever, this book offers a reassuring resource for parents who don't know how to start or where to turn for a helping hand.

chapter 1

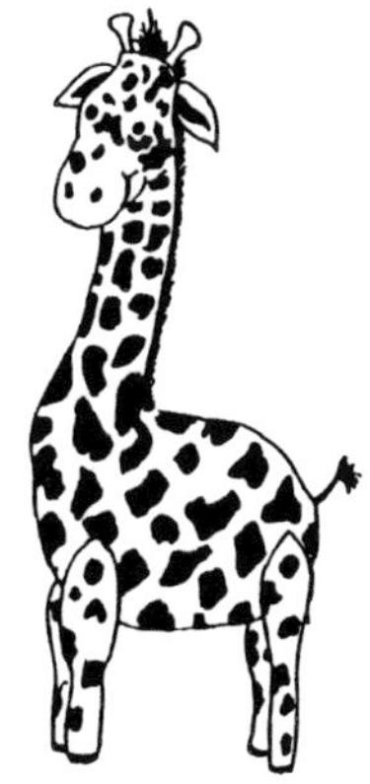

Can I afford in-home care or a day care center?

Listed below are some important questions for you and your family to consider before beginning the search for the right nanny or day care, center.

*1) Can you afford to pay someone without cutting back on other family activities?

*2) Is your schedule flexible enough to accommodate a stop at the day care en route to and/or from work?

*3) Does your work schedule require long hours, overtime, or traveling? Will your work directly affect your child care decision?

*4) Can friends or family fill in or help as needed? What would their help cost?

*5) Will you lose money if you stay home from work with a sick child? Might you be docked pay or even lose your job?

*6) Do you and your spouse's schedules overlap or are they identical? How do your schedules affect your child care needs?

GROUP DAY CARE:

Group day care is the choice most families rely on. When looking at group day care consider the following:

-There should be one teacher for every three or four babies age 2 or under, and/or one teacher for every five or six toddlers.

-The total number of children in a group should be small: no more than eight 2 year-olds or younger, no more than 12 toddlers.

-It must be possible for parents to check on children at the center. You should be able to drop by at any time and feel welcome, not feel like an intruder.

-The children should appear happy and active, not be wandering around aimlessly.

-Food should be nutritious and right for your child's dietary needs.

-The day care must have efficient arrangements for dealing with emergencies.

IN-HOME CHILD CARE:

Many two-income families choose to have one on one care in their own homes, rather than placing their children in day care. Unfortunately, nannies do not come cheap, and single parents often lack the option to choose in-home care. Day care fits their budgets better.

Parents who hire nannies are responsible not only for their salary but for their Social Security taxes and payroll deductions as well. The time spent keeping proper records can be considerable. On the plus side, there are Federal Income tax deductions for child care.

Beware of any household employee who requests to work for cash only. This sounds easy, but it can lead to trouble. If you do not take the proper taxes from an employee's salary, and the employee later seeks benefits from the government, she might get caught and be charged with fraud. This will also put you in a sticky situation. Not long ago my referral service was asked to appear in court and testify concerning a nanny who collected benefits from the government but had not reported all her earnings. Be cautious. Protect yourself from anyone who appears to be trying to cheat the government. You don't want to end up in court or have to be audited by the I.R.S.

If the cost of in-home care seems steep, check around at work. Some employers will offer compensation to help parents with the expense of in-home or day care. Enrolling in a dependent care flexible spending account program could reduce your taxable income by having money for child care taken out prior to taxes. Check with your employee benefits department to see if it offers such a program. Remember: child care for employees usually helps the employer. Not Always, of course.

Day care centers will not take a sick child and at any sign of illness, will call and ask the parent to pick the child up. Many employees miss occasional work days when their children attend day care center. If parents have nannies at home with their children, companies can usually count on fewer days missed and more work done.

Look at all your options when deciding what's right for your family, and compare the costs. Day care for one child under 2 costs around $100.00 a week. Some private home day cares are cheaper. A professional nanny for in-home care can cost from $200.00 to $400.00 a week but, if you can share a nanny, this cost may be split between two families.

chapter 2

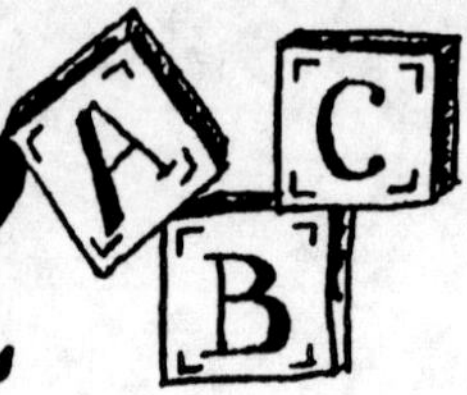

What kind of person do I need?

There are many kinds of in-home providers, and they go by different names and titles. The main ones with their job descriptions, are listed in paragraphs that follow. Look them over and you'll probably find the one which fits your family's needs.

Aide**- This means one who helps or furnishes, support, or relief for a family. She may be trained in basic medical training, like a nurse's aide.

American Au Pair **-("oh-pear") (American Style)-She lives with a family and provides help with household chores, taking care of the family's children part-time. She usually work under the direction of a parent, and may or may not have experience.

Au Pair**-("oh- pear") (European Style)- A European or other foreign national in the United States who does domestic work for a family in exchange for room and board, spending money, or the chance to learn a family's language and customs. She lives as part of the host family and receives a salary for doing household work and /or taking care of a child or children. Such individuals are not always experienced in child care or familiar with American children's needs. Be careful! Ask lots of questions about their culture and views on child discipline, before hiring. Many do not have previous experience in child care.

Caregiver**-A person who assists a sick or disabled person. One who attends to the needs of a child or dependent adult.

Caretaker**- One employed to look after or take charge of a person's property;a custodian.

Companion**-One who lives or travels with and assists a family in caring for a child or elderly person.

Domestic **-A housekeeper or servant who does household chores and errands.

Governess**-Traditionally, this is an educationally qualified person employed by a family for the full or part-time education of school age children. She only teaches and is not usually assigned either domestic work or the physical care of small children. Hours worked by a governess are agreed upon with the family. Sometimes a governess is employed to travel with a family and educate or train children on the move.

Helpmates **-They assist parents and act as an extension of the mother in performing duties of the home and caring for the family's children. They may live in or out.

Housekeeper**-One employed to perform or direct housekeeping.

House Sitter **-One who lives in and cares for a house while the family is away .

Housewife**-A woman managing her own household. A mother may often need help managing her home and/or children.

Live-in ** - Someone who resides at his or her place of employment, Such as a nanny or companion hired to take care of children or an elderly person.

Maid**- A person who is to take care of the household chores or housecleaning.

Mother's Helper **- One who assists a mother or family. A mother's helper could live-in or out and she works under direction of the family, but may be left temporarily with full responsibility for the children and or household.

Nanny**- A child's nurse, employed by a family on either a live-in or live-out basis exclusively for child care and domestic tasks. Solid character references are required for such a position. Nannies work different hours each week and are usually given total charge. Families should make a list of jobs to guide the nanny, to avoid any misunderstanding as to what's expected.

What does a nanny's job entail? She takes full charge of the family's children, including planning and preparing their meals. She manages the children's laundry, activities and outings, intellectual stimulation, language training, transportation, and discipline. Any housekeeping duties, that are child related. The nanny must be able to communicate with both parents and the children.

Who are nannies? They come in many shapes and sizes. They may be any age from eighteen to sixty. They should have a high school education,or the equivalent and be in good health, with up to date documentary proof of immunization and, as required, a negative TB test. Genuine love and respect for children is a must for nannies.

Nannies can be classified in three categories:

1) Single young women with day care and or baby-sitting experience. They want to work with children for a year or longer. A nanny of this description may have had prior jobs or have one at present. She wants to work closely with children for the satisfaction of giving this kind of one-on-one care.

2) Older and more mature women who have raised families and are drawn to in-home day care based on their past experience with children.

3) Women with a degree or educational background relating to children who want to work with a family to supplement classroom learning.

Nurse's Aide**- One who assist nurses at a medical facility or provides private care for a child or elderly person.

Nurse Practitioner**- A registered nurse with special training to care for sick or disabled children or adults. One employed to provide primary health care including many tasks customarily performed by a physician.

Nursery Nurse**-This title, used in Britain, refers to a person especially trained in young children's care. (but not limited to in-home care). When employed by a family , such nurses may live in or out. They work independently and are responsible for everything related to care of the children in their charge. Any domestic duties are generally related to the children. Besides specialized training, they must have successfully passed the National Certification Board Examination.

Sitter**-One who cares for babies, young children or adults when the parents or family aren't home. Elderly or disabled persons often need sitters.

Visiting Nurse **- This can be a registered nurse employed by a public health agency or hospital to promote community health, especially by visiting and treating sick people in their homes. One may be hired by a family to provide for private care for a child or elderly parent .

chapter 3

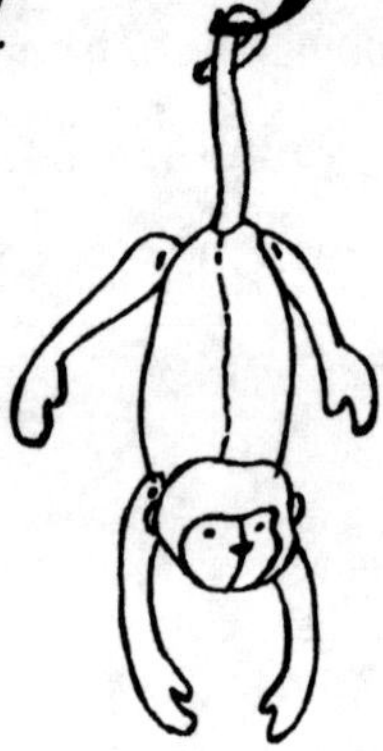

What's the job description? How long to find a helper?

How do you decide which of the many available helpers is for you? Well, look first at your family's needs and determine what hours must be worked. Prepare a realistic list of what duties the job will involve. Match these requirements as closely as possible to one of the descriptions in the previous chapter.

Be sure not to advertise for a nanny if it is really a housekeeper you need. Nannies are setting standards for themselves and striving for guidelines to follow in their field. A nanny will not be as good at cleaning as a housekeeper, and a housekeeper will not be as good at child care as a nanny. Training schools for nannies are becoming ever more popular. Nannies who are trained for positions in child care simply won't want a housekeeping job.

If you're a mother who will be at home, but needs backup, the job description for you is Mother's Helper. If you have to leave home regularly for short periods and just need someone to watch your child, you want a baby-sitter. While there is a growing demand for nannies, and some parents will only accept a nanny. Many sitters are experienced and well qualified to care for your children. A lot of caring people who love children and want to share this love find fulfillment as sitters.

Take time to find the right person and don't be rushed. Let any prospect stay with your child a while to see how they get along before you decide about hiring. Some caregivers, although experienced, may not be good for your child. If you rush, chances are you'll hire the wrong person. The key is to find someone compatible with your child. Children have their own personalities and preferences at an early age. Remember, if your child is not happy you won't be either.

The amount of time it will take to find someone who fits your need usually depends on work hours and requirements. If the job requirements are complicated or out of the ordinary, allow a bit more time to find the person with relevant experience. The time it will take to hire a person will also depend on the pay. Offer what the job is worth and you probably won't have to wait long for the right person.

Be thorough and methodical when interviewing.

Check all references and past work history carefully. This will go far toward preventing frequent turnovers of your household personnel. Allow a minimum of two to three weeks to screen all your prospects. Should you find a person you like who wants to start work earlier than you need someone, offer some part-time work until you are ready for a full-time helper. This will give you and your new helper a chance to ease the children into a changed situation more smoothly.

chapter 4

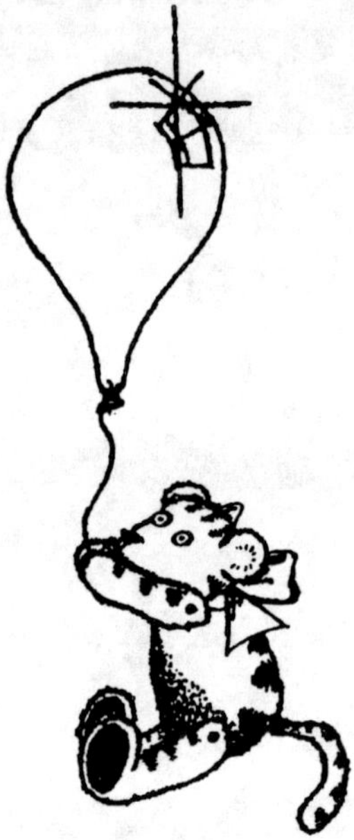

How do I check references and interview a caregiver?

You should require the following information when considering an applicant for a job in your home:

1) *Birth certificate*

2) *Social Security card.*

3) *Valid driver's license*

4) *A home phone number*

5) *A physical exam within the past two years.*

6) *Work references with addresses and phone numbers for the past three years.*

7) *Character references with addresses and phone numbers*

8) *Neighbor references and phone numbers.*

Mother's Helpmates referral service interviews both sitters and parents in their homes before making any final decision on placement. The technique of in-home interviewing helps us determine the character of all applicants and of those who live with them. We want to match the personalities of family and sitter. We can't risk placing a criminal or a potential child abuser or anyone who lives with such a person.

My interviewing technique is what makes our agency different from others. I always interview applicants in their homes. Most nannies don't mind, and it gives you a chance to get to know them in their own settings, and many feel more at ease during an interview at home. You can sometimes narrow down the applicants for a nanny position just by mentioning the in-home interview. Any applicants who have something to hide will change their mind about applying then and there. In case you feel apprehensive about going to an interview at someone's home alone, before having met the person, ask her to come to a restaurant or public place the first time. After narrowing the field, you can meet the best prospects at their homes to make a final decision.

Remember, the person you're seeking will be working in your home without any supervision. For this reason, I recommend interviewing any applicant you're seriously considering at least twice. The second time have the person come to your house for the interview, and have your children present to see her reaction to them and vice versa. Notice whether the nanny acknowledges or speaks to the children during the interview. Discuss your ideas for child rearing and disciplining and hers. Pay attention to her questions, as well as her answers. Make it clear that she should never discipline your children physically. Ask the applicant how she would handle a temper tantrum, and how she would handle some emergency.

Use examples from our application and screening sheet to check each applicant.. Don't skip over any important questions, and keep close track of all questions and answers. Always get the applicant's signature, without which you can't verify her previous employment and other information she provides. Review the information once more before the applicant leaves. Make sure the application sheet is filled out completely and signed.

The applicants appearance is always important. If a nanny or sitter doesn't look clean and neat before she has the job, she isn't likely to do so after being hired. After all, the person caring for your children will be responsible for keeping them clean and preparing their food. So now is the time to make judgments concerning appearance and personal hygiene.

When hiring someone, make copies of her Social Security card, birth certificate, driver's licence, and C.P.R. certificate. Keep these in a file on your employee. You may want to ask the applicants to make copies of these items and any other types of certifications they have, and bring them to the final interview. If you need someone with special training in caring for special-needs children, or for an elderly or disabled person, this is especially important.

MOTHER'S HELPMATES
RESEARCH &REFERRAL
APPLICATION FOR DOMESTIC/HOUSEHOLD

Name-First/ Middle /Last__________________S.S.#____/____/____
Address____________________City/State____________/Zip______
Spouse's Name- First/Middle/Last________________S.S.#___/__/__
Phone Home___________ / Work___________D.O.B.__________
Previous addresses for the last three years:____________________
____
Single-Married/Divorced/Separated-How many dependents do you have?
Are you an American citizen? yes>----no>— If not do you have a green card or visa to work in this country?—- Driver's License number#_____
Expiration date______ Has your license ever been revoked-?_________
Have you ever been convicted of a D.U.I.?______________________
Have you ever been in the military?____________Do you have your own transportation? Have you ever been convicted of a crime or do you live with someone who has been?_____Do you have any health problem that would interfere with your job?____Are you taking any medication?____
If you are applying for housekeeping have you ever been bonded or licensed?____ If so where and what is the company's phone number and address____
Have you ever been accused of child abuse either of your own children or someone else's?__________________Are you afraid of animals?____
Do you have a preference in religion?-----Do you smoke?___________
Do you prefer nonsmoking family?_____________________________
Would you submit to a drug screen?____________________________
Have you ever suffered from any kind of substance abuse?___________
How long have you lived in this state?__________________________
List any other states where you have lived and the addresses__________
____
Salary expected_______List three neighbors for character references who know you and or have lived next to you either now or in the past. Include their phone numbers and addresses:
(1)___________________________2)____________________________
3)___________________________4)____________________________

When was your last physical exam?________________________
Do you have any physical problems that would hinder your work?______
Whom do we contact in case of an emergency?_________________
Give a family member to contact.___________________________
What is the relationship of this person to you?_______________
Spouse's work #__________Do you have children?___________.
Your children's ages are?_________________If they were sick woulo you have someone to help care for them or would you have to miss work to take care of them?________ Educational background includes:_______
High school- grade finished_______Elementary__ grade finished______.
college or technical school training___________________________
List any special training___ Have you had C.P.R. or first aid training?__
____
Would you be willing to take C.P.R. training if asked to for the job?____
List three personal references including addresses and phone numbers:____
____
____
List your last employers including names and addresses and phone numbers:____
____
____
____
____
Work hours preferred are what shift?___________________________.
1st []___2nd[]__Overnight[]Available on Weekends?[] Will you work over 40 hours a week?____
How far do you live from the job?____________________________
What salary are you looking for?____What was your last salary? ______
Would you be willing to travel with the family or relocate if asked to? All the information on this application is true to the best of my knowledge. I understand if any criminal acts are found I can be discharged from my job immediately.

Signed:____.
Date:____

MOTHER'S HELPMATES
RESEARCH&REFERRAL
CHECK SHEET FOR INTERVIEWING
NANNY /COMPANION/ MOTHER'S HELPER

NAME____
PHONE——————DATE-__________TIME__________
POSITION BEING APPLIED FOR NANNY/COMPANION/
DOMESTIC/HOUSEKEEPER

COMMENTS-

[1]ON TIME____________________________________

[2]APPEARANCE ________________________________

[3]DURATION OF LAST JOB______________________

[4]STRONG POINTS ____________________________

[5]WORK ATTITUDE ____________________________

[6]WORK GOALS________________________________

[7] HOURS WANTED_____________________________

[8]TRANSPORTATION ___________________________

[9]CHARACTER_________________________________

[10]POSITIVE OR NEGATIVE_____________________

[11]RELIABILITY______________________________

[12]SALARY EXPECTED__________________________

[13]EXPERIENCE_______________________________
Notes____
____

(1) MOTHER'S HELPMATES REFERRAL APPLICATION FOR NANNY/COMPANION

Name ________________ S.S.#:__________ Date__________

Address:________________________________

City/State______________ Zip:______________ Race:__________

Home phone no———Daytime no:——— U.S.citizen __________

How long have you lived at this address ?________________

If less than 3 years attach a list of all addresses for the past 3 years.

Height __________ Weight __________ Hair color __________ Eye color ____

Date of birth: / / Drivers licence no. : __________ State ______

Number of children/persons willing to sit with?______________

Available on Week -ends?__________ Hours?__________

Will you sit with handicapped person, elderly person, people and/or children?

____

Are you willing to clean or cook if asked?________________

Preference in religion?________________________

Would you submit to a drug screen?________Have you ever been convicted of a crime?__________ Have you ever been bonded or licensed? Yes____No__

Do you smoke?______Do you drink?________________Do you prefer non-smoker family?____________________

Do you have transportation?______________Do you have a copy of your Birth certificate?__Are you willing to attend classes for your job?________

What salary do you expect to be paid?______________

(2)

Have you ever been accused of abuse to a child or adult?_______________

Will you take any classes which this job may require? Like taking C.P.R?____

Have you ever suffered from substance or alcohol abuse?_______________

List all personal references you can supply (include addresses and phone numbers:_______________________________________
____
____
____

List all education and training (attach copies of the certificates and resume):____
____

References must be checked before being placed._______________

- List any information that will help:_______________________________
____
____

My hobbies:_______________________________________
Do you have any health problems that would hinder your work?_______________
Are you pregnant? _______________________________
Have you had physical in the past two years:________ Person to call in case of an emergency:_______________________________
Additional information:_______________________________
To the best of my knowledge, all my information is true and listed._______________

- Sign__________________________Date__________________________
- I understand if I supply any falsified information I can be dismissed from my job by the family at that time._______________________________
- Special notes or request_______________________________________
- ____
- ____
- ____

chapter 5

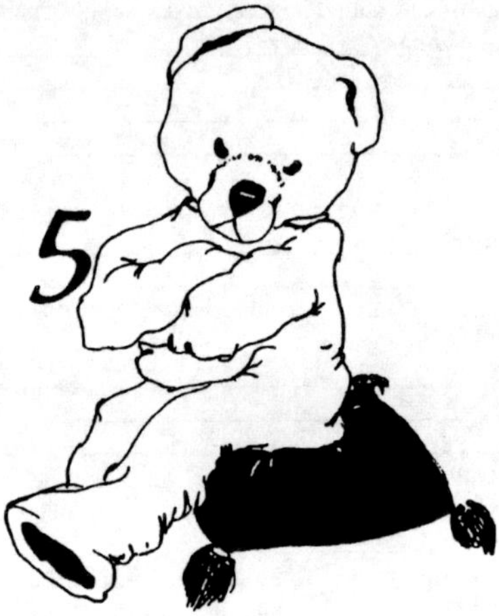

How do I keep my nanny when she's the right one?

The question I am asked most often after placing a nanny is, "How can I make her stay with my family forever?" Most parents expect their nanny, housekeeper, or sitter to do everything- -but they also expect to pay a minimum wage. Of course, some parents cannot afford to pay much, especially those who are single. Ironically, though, the family that makes less money usually offers to pay their nanny the most. Families that have more to offer are seldom fair when deciding a salary. Ask yourself, "Would I do this job for this amount of money?" If your answer is no, then reconsider. After all, if you won't do it, what makes you think someone else will?

When you start interviewing applicants, you will find that nannies and housekeepers are looking for better paying jobs than in the past. The pay an applicant is offered should recognize past experience in child care or elderly care. Nannies are not going to stay long on a job that pays $4.00 or $5.00 an hour if they hear that someone else is paying more for similar work.

The more competitive the pay, you offer the

longer a nanny will stay. Before I place a nanny in a home, I look at the family's past history with nannies. Families that offer low pay and poor treatment of their nannies have a high turnover. If you want a nanny to stay, look carefully at what pay you are offering. Do you offer the going rate of pay for the area where you live? You can find this rate by calling the nanny or placement agencies in your town. Never offer a low rate if you are serious about finding and keeping a nanny.

The extent of experience a nanny has in child care must always be taken in to consideration. An educated nanny will want top salary and will look for a family that offers this pay. Some nannies in urgent need of a job may accept a smaller salary also when offered such extras as: room and board or the use of a vehicle. In some cases, you might want to offer a nanny such compensation in kind along with lower salary. Allowing a nanny to live-in during the work week will save her the cost of transportation to and from her job. A lower salary may be easier to negotiate if her outside expenses can be cut.

If you want a nanny to stay with your family,

don't hire one who has jumped from job to job. Chances are this nanny will not be with you for long. Also, if a nanny has traveled a lot, there is less chance of her staying with you. A local nanny is a better choice because she more likely wants to stay in the area.

Respect your nanny's days off. A sure way to lose a nanny is not to allow her enough free time. Nannies are people, too. Besides, they will do a better job when they get sufficient rest. A nanny or companion should have at least two days of recuperation a week. Don't think that because you have a live-in she is always at your beck and call. Some families that hire live-ins, seem to have the misconception that a nanny should work 24 hours a day for eight hours pay. Families who request such long hour's should be reminded that slavery is against the law. No one wants to work all the time.

A new mother who has had a caesarean, or has a colicky baby, may need a nanny around the clock. The typical solution is to schedule more than one nanny to give each one some time off. The work hours for any live-in should stay as close to a permanent schedule as possible. This will enable her to schedule her own activities and take care of personal business.

Live-in nannies are the hardest for families to keep because they usually don't get enough time off. They burn out fast and quit. Families who work long hours may request a live-in because of their erratic schedules. This is often true of doctors, or parents whose jobs involve traveling. Elderly or disabled persons who cannot care for themselves also need live-ins for around the clock help. When this is the case, there should be three shifts of sitters or nurses giving such care.

Overtime is another problem. Compensate your nanny for any time worked beyond normal duty hours. Do not expect her to work extra hours without reward. Nannies realize there are times when you need them for overtime work, but they deserve appreciation for their extra efforts. Lack of appreciation is another complaint often heard from a sitters who are quitting. If they do their job well or go out of their way for you show your appreciation by thanking them warmly. Remember, they take care of the most important persons in your home.

Always pay your helper as promised; don't

be late with pay. She needs money for her bills just as you do for yours. And another thing: Make sure your nanny's surroundings are comfortable. Ask yourself if you would be comfortable in her place. You should feel good about the surroundings you offer her to work in. If you need a live-in, make sure you have adequate accommodations, including a private bathroom and bedroom. Not being respected is a another complaint of unhappy nannies. Don't treat them as if they're beneath you. Treat them with the respect you would want yourself. I often hear people say, "I just want someone who can follow instruction. I don't want a nanny to be my friend. " But I think they <u>should</u> want the nanny be their friend and to feel like part of the family.

Good communication will help build a lasting relationship with your nanny or caregiver. Be sure to explain what her duties are and what you expect. Don't ever assume the nanny just knows! Make a list of your instructions to avoid misunderstandings, but don't put so much on the list that its impossible to get everything done on time. Parents often complain that their nanny isn't doing what they want. Most of the time, the problem is she doesn't have a clue as to what they want. When this happens, it's time for nanny and family to sit down and talk and to make that list if there isn't one.

Nannies aren't mind readers. So don't assume they will do a job the same way you do. There are different ways to clean and still get the job done. Some parents say, "I'm paying her to do things my way." Wrong! Try to compromise. What difference does it make how it's done as long as the job gets done?

Don't compare your present nanny to a previous one. The new nanny doesn't want to hear that she will never take the place of the last one. No two people and nannies are ever alike. Discuss your own ideas on child rearing and discipline with her and compare your own similarities and differences. But not those of other nannies.

When hiring a nanny, look at her religious beliefs and ask yourself whether they conflict with your own. Consider her lifestyle, past and present. If something bothers you, don't hire the woman only to dismiss her a little later. Nannies are not going to change their ideas or their way of life for a job. Go over their character references and comments, and don't hire someone who doesn't seem to have good morals. The time to talk and find out about these important issues is before, not after, you hire your nanny.

Here are some things to explore. Does she have a fiancee or husband? Do they have children? Who will stay home and take care of them when they are sick? How soon do they want to start a family? Find out if your applicant is a student in school or is planning to go back to school in the future. Don't hire a student who is plans to return to school after only a short time on the job. Her student schedule may interfere with your working hours, forcing you to replace her sooner or later.

There are several important things to consider when hiring a middle-aged or older, nanny. Older nannies have more experience, but they may also have more problems about taking instructions. Most of them don't know how to swim or know C.P.R. Consider such problems as these when you are interviewing a nanny. Children love water, whether they can swim or not, and they can easily fall in. If a nanny is afraid of the water or can't swim you should not employ her. Even children who know how to swim may have accidents and need help. Lack of C.P.R training is another problem I run into often when interviewing and working with older nannies. Some believe that because they raised their own children without the use a of C.P.R, they shouldn't have to start now. Many resent being given any instructions at all about child rearing, especially if they have grown children of their own.

Make sure to ask every applicant the questions we have discussed in this and the previous chapter and to take careful note of the responses. A parent must feel comfortable about leaving a nanny in charge of household and children. I've been told by some older nannies." I know how to take control of children. Families have to respect what I say or I leave". To avoid buying problems with attitudes like this, dig out the nanny's attitudes toward her job when you interview her, and save the trouble of replacing her later.

chapter 6

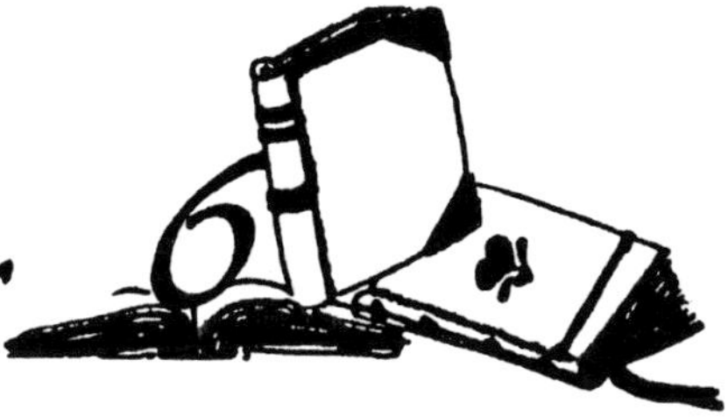

What do I pay a nanny?

Salary depends on the job to be done and the amount of experience an applicant has. Average hourly wages vary between $5.00 and $10.00 in most states. Consider the cost of living in your area. For example, wages are higher in Boston than in Tampa. One way to find out what's fair market is to ask someone who employs a nanny or sitter. Or call a few agencies listed in the yellow pages under child care and see what they can tell you. When asking about the wage, give the job description.

If you are serious about hiring someone, don't offer low-end wages. I often hear complaints from nannies who have been offered ridiculously low pay. Make sure you can afford a nanny's salary before you ever start to advertise for one. You don't want to advertise and then find out the going rate is higher than you can pay.

If some applicant asks for a very small salary, be suspicious. The sitter may have a criminal record and be looking for work with unsuspecting parents in such a hurry to find a nanny that they overlook such details. Or parents who can ill afford a high salary, and think a nanny who accepts a pittance is a good deal. This could spell trouble. Watch out for such people. Your child's safety may be at risk.

Discuss with the nanny the amount of her salary after taxes are withheld. Make sure she is clear on what she will actually be paid. We will discuss withholding taxes in chapter 9. If the nanny depends on a certain income, she may need to know the exact amount she will be paid. Discuss also what benefits you can and can't offer. There may be unemployment taxes you will need to consider along with her salary, and other payroll deductions. If the sitter wants to be paid cash, make sure she understands she is responsible for paying her own taxes, assuming she is self-employed.

It is usually a good idea to put together your own parent-and-nanny contract and to have your new employee sign it. (See the example later in this chapter). If your nanny is an independent contractor working for herself, you may be able to give her a 1099 at year's end. Keep close track of all salary you pay your nanny.

Here are some suggestions about different pay

situations:

Live-in salaries These should include any extra expenses paid for utilities and food along with the weekly salary.

Sharing a nanny Some nannies or companions work for several families on a short-term basis, taking job leads from referral and home health agencies. Their weekly salary is to be split between the employing families. The hourly rate for such a nanny may be a little higher, to compensate for the strain of caring for more than one child at more than one house.

Housekeeper salaries are usually $10.00 an hour. If the employee is a nanny or sitter, the hourly rate will range from $5.00 and $8.00 an hour.

Maids and cleaning service personnel get an average of $10.00 an hour.

Holiday and vacation pay should be discussed in advance with your nanny. Families that get holiday and vacation pay themselves should offer these benefits to their nanny. The nanny can be off during the same holidays and vacation periods as the family. Some families may want to require a probation period before offering any such benefits.

Insurance is usually offered by families that can afford this for their employee, although most families will probably feel they can't afford it . When everything is put in writing there are less misunderstandings about salary and duties are minimized.

INDEPENDENT CONTRACTING AGREEMENT

______________________________, referred to as CONTRACTING PARTY, and ______________________________, referred to as INDEPENDENT CONTRACTOR, agree:

INDEPENDENT CONTRACTOR shall perform the following services for CONTRACTING PARTY:

____

at the following rate of remuneration:

____

This agreement shall begin on ________________________ and shall terminate on ________________________ unless earlier terminated.

Contracting Party may terminate this contract on 14 days notice to Independent Contractor for unsatisfactory performance.

THIS IS AN AGREEMENT FOR INDEPENDENT CONTRACTING SERVICES. THE CONTRACTING PARTY PROVIDES NO BENEFITS SUCH AS UNEMPLOYMENT INSURANCE, HEALTH INSURANCE OR WORKER'S COMPENSATION INSURANCE TO INDEPENDENT CONTRACTOR.

CONTRACTING PARTY IS ONLY INTERESTED IN THE RESULTS OBTAINED BY THE INDEPENDENT CONTRACTOR. INDEPENDENT CONTRACTOR SHALL BE RESPONSIBLE FOR PROVIDING ALL TOOLS AND MATERIALS REQUIRED FOR PERFORMANCE OF THE TASKS AGREED TO.

INDEPENDENT CONTRACTOR IS RESPONSIBLE FOR PAYMENT OF ALL FEDERAL, STATE AND LOCAL INCOME TAXES.

Dated: ____________________________

____

CONTRACTING PARTY BY AN AUTHORIZED OFFICER

____

INDEPENDENT CONTRACTOR

Parent and Nanny Agreement

Agreement between employers)——and———(employee).

1.This agreement covers the time period from Date—to—

2. Termination of agreement:

(A.) If the employee is terminated for cause,the employer is not bound to this agreement; however one week's severance pay will be given. After the employee has worked—- months.

(B.) If the employee decides to leave the position, the employee will provide at least three weeks notice. No severance pay is required if the employer wishes to terminate before the three-week period.

(C.) At the time of employee's termination, any outstanding bills incurred by the employer on behalf of the employee may be deducted from the employee's pay.

3.This agreement (and any part thereof) may be amended at any time with the mutual agreement and signature of all parties.

4.Review of agreement, performance, and salary set for the following dates .Quarterly or etc.

Date:————-Date:——-Date:———

5.This full time child care position includes but is not limited to the following responsibilities:

A. To provide child care up to— hours per day

B. To provide "light housekeeping", which means any child care- related duties (i. e. preparing formula , cleaning up after feeding, children's laundry, etc.)

C. To use creative skills in planning activities that promote the physical, emotional, intellectual and social development of the child, as approved by the parent or guardian.

D. To comply with parent's discipline and child rearing preferences.

E. To maintain a cheerful and helpful attitude while on duty
F. To promote feelings of security and warmth by planning daily cuddle/reading/talk time with each child.
G. To write daily log sheets of events and to confer with parents about special problems, child's newly learned skills, etc., so as to promote good communication with parents concerning child's daytime life.
H. To provide reasonable flexibility in time of emergency or unexpected schedule changes.
I. To read/ review any pertinent literature provided by parents in order to promote broader knowledge of child rearing philosophy, education and/or child psychology.

6. Additional responsibilities:

* Children's bedroom and playroom picked up and crib sheets changed once per week.
*Vacuuming of the children's bedroom and playroom once per week.
* Empty diaper pail into garage trash cans daily.
*Prepare formula bottles as needed.
*Provide children with a minimum of two hours of fresh air daily, weather permitting.
*Bathe each child as needed or if requested by parent.
* Load, unload and run dishwasher as needed.
*Feed pets daily.
*Occasionally do parent laundry.
*Occasionally defrost and/or begin preparation of parent dinner.

7 .Transporting children:

Children are not to be transported anywhere without permission of parents.

8. Work schedule:

Monday through Friday — a.m. to— p.m. or up to hours per day with the total not to exceed 50 hours per week.

9. Compensation:

A. Employers agree to pay the employee a base salary of $——per week from date———-until date——-and then to pay $——per week beginning (Date:———-)

B. Salary is to be paid every week on Friday covering the period of Monday through Friday of the previous week. First week's salary will be withheld.

C. Overtime compensation is paid at a rate of $——per hour or at 1 and 1/2 times the hourly rate of current salary.

10. Taxes:

A. The employer will take out the appropriate taxes and social security from the employee's salary.

B. If the employee is an independent contractor she is responsible to report all earned income and to pay all appropriates taxes . Employee will be given a Form 1099.

11. Vacation:

Employers agree to allow the employee one week of vacation to be taken after six or twelve months of employment.

Employer______________Employer________Date:____

Employee______________Date:__________________

chapter 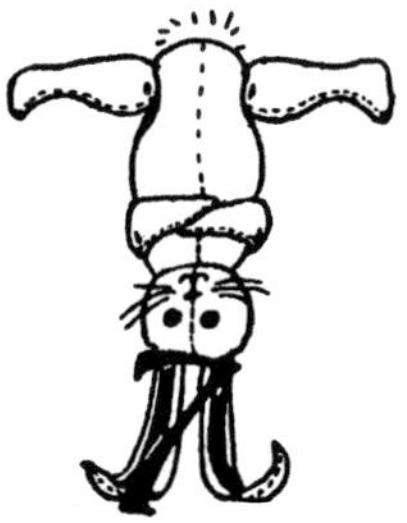

Where do I find a helpmate? How do I advertise?

The first step in advertising for a nanny is to have the right job description. Be precise in your ad. Keep it short. Advertising in the major newspapers can be expensive, so place ads in the community shopper guides. Smaller community papers offer cheaper advertising and your applicants will be closer to where you live. Call your church and community services and ask if they have bulletin boards for posting help wanted ads. Call the YMCA for a list of private in-home day cares in your area. The YMCA has a child care referral service to help parents find sitters, nanny placement services, and day care centers in your area. You can also go to any community college in your area and place ads on the bulletin boards there for students who are looking for jobs. Put your ads near the school's Early Childhood Education Department. Students there are perfect candidates because they are interested in working with children. Look in the yellow pages for any nanny schools (and check our list of nanny schools in this book.) Such schools have nannies available for families to hire. If you do not find any nanny schools in the yellow pages, call your library for any listings it has in your area. Radio stations offer community service announcements, so why not ask the station to announce your job? Nursing schools always have students studying pediatric nursing or certified nursing assistants who are looking for work. These women are trained and qualified to help families with normal or special-needs children and disabled persons. Nursing schools also have information on C.P. R. classes, in case you want your sitter or nanny to be certified in C.P.R. or first aid.

Another source for nanny applicants is Senior Neighbors services in your area. Ask if they know of any senior citizens who want part time work for extra income. Keep in mind that some senior citizens may not have the energy to handle toddlers, but this will depend on the individual. Senior citizens can sit with a sick loved one or with a disabled child. Make sure, if you have a swimming pool, that any older person you hire is not afraid of water and can swim, in case your child falls in. When you call Senior Neighbors pass on all the pertinent information about the job you're offering, such as whether you have pets, a pool, etc.

Pets, whether in or outside the home, should be mentioned in your advertisement, in case applicants may have allergies or a fear of dogs. Mention any "special" pets, like snakes or other unusual animals. Below are some examples of ads and an outline of the things to mention when putting your ad together:

(a) The job description

(b) The location of the job

(c) Weekly salary or hourly rate

(d) Days of the week

(e) Experience or special training needed for the job.

(f) Transportation needed or available

Sitter Needed From (7:00 - 8:00 A.M) to (3:00 - 5:00 P.M) M-F Near Rossville Area Must Have Reliable Transportation to Transport Children to and From School /Nonsmoker/ References Required. (Call 555-1234) After 4:00 Family Has Dog $6.00 An Hour

Here's a sample ad:

Domestic Help Wanted to Clean/Cook Do Laundry
Mondays & Saturdays 12 P.M. to 3 P.M. $7.50 An Hour
Call Beeper No. .347-0987

And Another

NEEDED:

Live-in Companion For Special Needs Child. Must be C.N.A.(Mon.- Fri.)$300.00 A Week/Benefits/ Nonsmoker/References Checked/Phone 555-1234

And still another:

(When putting an ad together for a bulletin board at a church or school, make it colorful to attract the attention of all passersby.)

ATTENTION

NEEDED: House sitter For Two Weeks Duties Include: Care of Family's Pet Cat and Gold Fish. Water Plants, Collect Mail, Salary is $150.00 for Two weeks/ Must Have Local References If Interested Call Betty at 555-1234

ATTENTION:

NEEDED SITTER FOR IN -HOME
CARE FOR NEWBORN . JOB LOCATION IS NEAR
HILLSBOROUGH BLVD. MUST HAVE
LOTS OF LOVE FOR CHILDREN
EXPERIENCE - REFERENCES- TRANSPORTATION
MON.-FRI. 8:00 AM TO 5:00
PAY IS $5.00 AN HOUR
CONTACT PASTOR JONES
OR CALL (555-1224)

all the community college and ask for student affairs or send or fax to this office your ad for posting on a bulletin board. A sample fax cover sheet follows:

ATTENTION: Student services/ John Smith

Jane Hill Campus

Fax no 222-444

From Mary Jo Thomas 222-3333

Fax no. 555-1234

Mr. Smith, here is a job bulletin to post at the school for the job we discussed Friday. If there are any questions please call/ or have all applicants call 222-5555 or fax me their resume .

I thank you for your help.

Thank You!

Sincerely,

Mrs. Thomas

Here's another example of an ad for a bulletin board.

ATTENTION:
MARY JO SMITH IS LOOKING FOR A
LOVING NANNY FOR HER TWO CHILDREN
FOR AFTER SCHOOL MONDAY- FRIDAY HOURS
PAY IS $5.25 PLUS MILEAGE/ HOURS ARE 2:00 TO
7:00 PM DUTIES INCLUDE:
PICKING THE CHILDREN UP AT SCHOOL. SOME
LIGHT HOUSEKEEPING PREPARE MEALS FOR
CHILDREN.
THE FOLLOWING IS NEEDED
EXPERIENCE/REFERENCES/RELIABLE
TRANSPORTATION/HOME PHONE.
IF INTERESTED PLEASE CALL 222-3333
OR FAX RESUME TO 555-1234

chapter 8

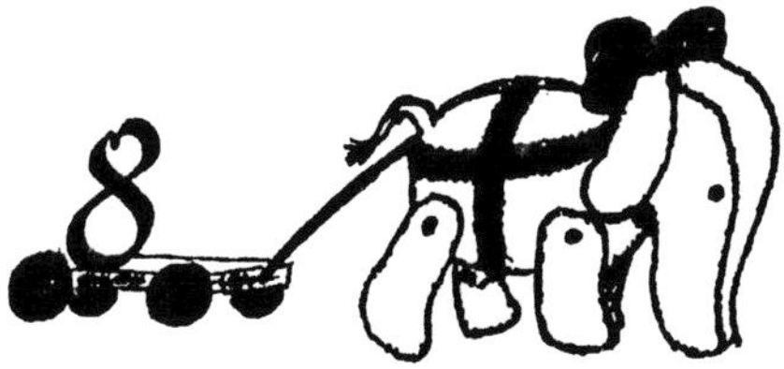

Screening your household help.

It is important for you as an employer to screen any employee. It is even more important to screen the person who is going to provide child care in your home. This chapter deals with the ins and outs of the screening process. In order for you to screen someone properly without the assistance of an agency, you will need the full cooperation of your potential nanny or housekeeper. This chapter will also show you how to get help from professional services that offer employee screening for employers.

The following are some areas to look closely at when screening employees yourself:

Past employment history- Look at the duration of the applicant's past jobs. This can help you to assess the amount of commitment they have. If their past jobs were mostly short- term, find out why. Did the family move, or were they hired only for a short period? Get the phone numbers and addresses of the previous employers and then call them to check the references. You can also write for further information using a Performance Request Form such as the one included toward the end of this chapter, after the section on Character References. You may get a more detailed reference by sending such a check list. Criminal Background: You will want to do a check for any criminal background. This can be done in a number of ways. One way is to get a release form signed by the applicant enabling you to query the appropriate authorities. An example of a release form is included at the end of this chapter. Alternatively, you can have the nanny obtain a copy of her own record for you or have her ask that one be sent to you. You may want to call a pre-employment screening service which, for a small fee, will do the screening for you. Paralegal and detective services offer pre-employment checks and can save you a lot of time screening a nanny. If the applicant has had a number of jobs outside your state, you will probably want to have an agency do the screening. It would have easy access to information that a private individual could not obtain without a hassle. You can find phone numbers for the above types of organizations in the yellow pages.

Although it's not easy to conduct the checks by yourself, it can save you some money if you have time to do so. Another way to get information on someone's criminal background is to write or call the F.BI's Identification Department in Washington, DC, at 1-202-324-5278. They can direct you to the agency in your state that will provide criminal background information on caregivers. When calling the F.BI, explain why you are asking for such criminal background data. Tell them you want to protect your child from any criminal or child abuser. They will be glad to help you contact the proper agency.

Abuse Registries are available in many states that record complaint reports of child abuse. A new law passed along with the Brady bill, called the National Child Protection Act of 1993 (Public Law 103-209- Dec. 20,1993), will make it easier to keep track of child abusers all over the country.

This law requires each state to report all child abuse information to a national child abuse records system established in Washington, DC.

Each state is also empowered to pass legislation which requires employers and agencies to contact a state agency and request a nationwide background check for the purpose of determining whether a provider has been convicted of a crime that bears upon his or her fitness to have responsibility for the safety and well-being of children.

The state agency shall access and review state and Federal criminal history through the national criminal history background check system and make reasonable efforts to respond to any inquiry within 15 business days.

Any background check will be handled in accordance with requirements of Public Law 92-544.

The law pertains to any business or organization whether public, private, for non-profit, for profit or voluntary, that provides child care or child care placement services, including a business or organization that licenses or certifies others to provide child care or child care placement services.

The child care abuse information reported by each state will contain the following facts: on persons who have been arrested for, or has been convicted of child abuse crime: full name, race, sex, date of birth, height, weight, fingerprints, a brief description of the child abuse crime or offenses for which the person has been arrested or convicted, the disposition of the charge, and any other information that the Attorney General deems useful in identifying persons arrested for, or convicted of, a child abuse crime.

For more complete information on The National Child Protection Act, call or write to:

> Federal Bureau of Investigation
> National Crime Information Center
> 10th and Pennsylvania Avenue, N.W.
> Washington, DC 20535

The following pages list various state agencies throughout the country which can help you obtain criminal background information. Here is one final thought, however, before you start this process by yourself. It will take a lot of time to get the information you need. Especially if the nanny or caregiver has lived in several states, it will be much easier to use an agency. Besides saving time, you'll save the cost of many long-distance phone calls.

Here are some numbers to call for information on obtaining a criminal background check in your state:

Alabama- Alabama State Human Services 205-298-7882
Alabama- Alabama State Patrol 205-865-3451
Alaska State Troopers-907-766-2552
Alaska State Troopers-907-438-2019
Arizona State Government - 602-921-4400
Arizona Law Enforcement- 602-223-2515
Arkansas Highway Patrol- 501-247-1483
California State Police-916-445-1150
Colorado State Highway-303-824-5010
Connecticut State Police-203-347-4333
Connecticut State Police-203-623-3634
Delaware State Police Troop- 302-577-3008
Delaware State Police Troop- 302-577-3051
Florida Department of Law Enforcement- 904-488-5081

Georgia Criminal Information Department-
404-244-2601
Georgia State Human Resource- 404-358-2657
Hawaii State Police-808-732-0727
Illinois Criminal Justice Department- 312-793-8550
Indiana State Police-219-636-2262
Iowa State Patrol-319-385-8715
Kansas State Highway Department-316-723-2503
Kentucky State Police-502-826-3312
Louisiana Criminal Justice Department-504-922-6095
Louisiana State Police- 504-295-8500
Maine State Police- 207-793-4500
Maryland State Police-410-486-3101
Massachusetts Department of Public Safety -
617-566-4500
Michigan State Police-517-362-3434
Michigan State transportation Department-
616-979-1170
Minnesota Department of Public Safety -
612-642-0670
Missouri Highway Patrol- 314-751-3313
Mississippi State Government -601-939-8640
Montana State Highway Patrol-406-365-5238
Nebraska State Patrol - 402-475-4545
Nevada Highway Patrol-702-486-4100
New Hampshire State Police-603-846-5517
New Hampshire Safety Department- 603-358-3333
New Jersey State Department-609-292-2121
New Jersey Criminal Justice Department-
609-984-6500
New Mexico State Government-505-461-1206
New York Department of Justice - 518-457-6113

North Carolina State Patrol- 919-747-2420
North Carolina State Government-919-274-1681
North Dakota Highway Patrol- 701-774-4360
North Dakota Human Service- 701-255-3090
Ohio State Police-419-826-5871
Ohio State Police-419-599-0991
Oklahoma State Highway Patrol-918-968-3000
Oklahoma State Highway- 405-258-0494
Oregon State Department of Police Public Service- 503-378-3720
Pennsylvania State Patrol - 717-783-5588
Rhode Island State Police-401-846-8200
Rhode Island Sheriffs Office- 401- 841-8300
South Carolina State Highway Patrol-803-874-4141
South Carolina State Patrol-803-882-5679
South Dakota-State Patrol-605-339-6601
Tennessee Sheriffs Office - 615-862-8123
Texas Criminal justice Department - 512-465-2151 or 512-463-9988 or 512-463-0345
Utah State Government-801-752-2511
Utah State Human Service -801-586-3841
Utah State Highway Patrol-801-654-2073
Vermont State Police Beheld-802-234-9933
Vermont State police Enosburg- 802-933-5555
Virginia State Police-804-674-2000
Washington DC Criminal Justice - 202-324-5278
West Virginia State Police- 304-843-4100
West Virginia State Police-304-824-5798
Wisconsin State Patrol- 608-269-2500
Wisconsin State Patrol- 715-386-3248
Wyoming State Patrol-307-754-3666
Wyoming State Government--307-469-2234

An example of a criminal background release form for you to use when requesting criminal background information follows:

(Name and address of person requesting the information)
Jane Smith
324 East Strawberry Ave
Chattanooga, Tennessee
37415

Jane Smith is requesting a criminal background release on the individual named below to be employed by our family for the care of our children .

DATE:____________________
NAME:____________________
D.O.B:____________________
RACE:____________________
S.S.#:____________________

All alias names used:(such as all maiden or married names used by employee.) ____________________

I understand and agree to any criminal background check for the benefit of the individual named above.

I____________________ give permission and agree by my signature to releasing any and all such information to Jane Smith.

____

Applicants

____

Employer

<u>Character references-</u> You should always get applicant character references. These may be checked by sending the character reference form to, or by calling, the references provided. Ask for their insight into the applicant's character. If possible, have them sign a release form releasing for your use all their information on the nanny's past work history. You'll find an example of the form to use on the following page.

EMPLOYMENT PERFORMANCE
REQUEST FORM

(*Applicant's name*)____________________has applied for work in our home.

The nanny or housekeeper has listed you as an employer from *date* to *date*. We would appreciate you answering these questions on *applicant first name* work performance. Thank you!

Name of former employer_________________________

Address_____________City/State/Zip_____________

Previous salary________________ Reasons for leaving?

____

Would you hire this person again to work for your family?____

Please check below:

Work quality was- Good ☐ Fair ☐ Excellent ☐

Job attitude was- Good Fair ☐ Excellent ☐

Was the employee on time?____ Always ☐ Sometimes ☐

Never ☐

If there were problems with the employee's work please state the reasons and circumstances.________________

List any additional information that could help us in our decision .______________________________________

____

Prospective Employer's Signature__________________

Date:______________________

EMPLOYMENT AND CHARACTER REFERENCE RELEASE FORM

List your past employers below along with their addresses and phone numbers.

Name of employer or family:______________________________

Address________________City/State/Zip_________Phone_________

Number of children in your care and their ages.____________Reasons for leaving:______________________________

Name of employer or family:______________________________

Address:________________City/State/Zip/________Phone_________

Number of children in your care and their ages____________Reasons for leaving :______________________________

Salary paid:_____________

Name of employer or family:________________Address:__________

____________________City/State/Zip______________Phone:____

Number of children in your care and their ages.____________Reasons for leaving:________________________________Salary paid:________

Please name at lease three character reference.

Please list the names addresses and phone numbers of these persons you have known for one year or more.

Name ___________________Address_______City/State/Zip________

Phone________________Known from______to________________

Name___________________Address________City/State/Zip_______

Phone________________Known from______to________________

Name___________________Address_______City/State/Zip________

Phone________________Known from______to________________

The facts I have listed are true. By my signature I give my permission to release any information as to my personal, employment or credit history to the person requesting. I understand that if any information above is false I can lose my job immediately.

Signature__________________________Date:__________________

Driving record: You will want to check an applicant's driving record to see if there is any history of driving infractions. You should know about any past D.U.I. (Driving Under the Influence of alcohol) violations, speeding tickets, or accidents. This is important information if the applicant is going to be driving your children to and from school or other activities. To get a copy of someone's driving record you'll need to provide the following identification data:

His or her full name, all residences during past years, date of birth, driver's license number, and social security number. You may make your request in person or write to your Department of Motor Vehicles. In most states you can also call the Highway Patrol for such information. The cost for obtaining this driving record is between $3.00 to $5.00 for the first page, with each additional page usually costing $1.00. When requesting the record by mail, you'll need to send the identifying data to the Department of Motor Vehicles or the Clerk of the Circuit Court and specifically request the person's driving record. You can also call for a request form, which they will send you to fill out and return. A notarized letter explaining why you are requesting the driving record, may also be helpful. Don't forget to include any fees that are applicable.

Credit report: You might want to check an applicant's credit to see whether they've any history of writing bad checks or have had any addresses (revealed by the credit report) besides those listed on the application. Most families won't care whether the employee has "good" credit. This check is just another precautionary step aimed at protecting your home and child from a potential thief.

Check on education and training: Some applicants will give a list of special training to impress you with their qualifications. You may want to verify such information, especially if this special training is in fact needed for care of your child or a handicapped person. To do this get the name and address of school(s) they claim to have attended and query these schools. Also check with the state to verify any nursing or nursing assistant certifications. Nannies and sitters do not, on the average, have a lot of education or job experience except in child care. The only qualifications a nanny really needs are to have good character and lots of love for children.

Physical exam or drug testing- The person should have had a recent physical exam(within the past two years). You want someone who is healthy enough to care for your child. Make sure the applicant is not taking any drugs or medications that will hinder taking care of your child. A physical exam is one way to check for drug abuse. You may have your family doctor set up the examination and you should pay for all costs. Be sure to get the applicants permission to receive the results of the examination.

chapter 9

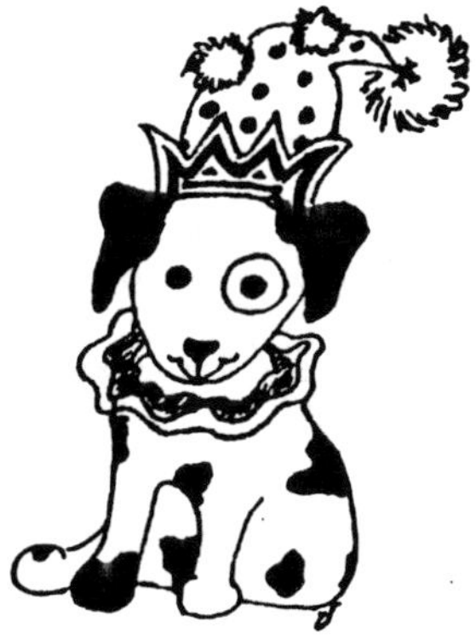

Taxes, Social Security and payroll programs

In this chapter we will discuss tax laws, Social Security taxes, unemployment taxes, and payroll arrangements for your household employee. When you hire domestic help, you have to comply with certain tax laws. This chapter explains your tax responsibilities as an employer. As you might have heard, even prominent U.S. government officials have failed to pay Social Security taxes on their employees and incurred heavy penalties as a result. Don't let ignorance cause you similar problems. Parents must know the tax responsibilities they assume by employing domestic help. An important fact is that you are not responsible in regard to the taxes of a person who is "self-employed". You may want to give an independent contract to any such person making this clear. The following pages outline different forms to use for your employee taxes and child care tax deductions.

□ S.S.-4 Application for employer identification number.-When you hire someone you will need to submit one of these.

Form **SS-4**
(Rev. December 1993)
Department of the Treasury
Internal Revenue Service

Application for Employer Identification Number

(For use by employers, corporations, partnerships, trusts, estates, churches, government agencies, certain individuals, and others. See instructions.)

EIN

OMB No. 1545-0003
Expires 12-31-96

Please type or print clearly.

1 Name of applicant (Legal name) (See instructions.)

2 Trade name of business, if different from name in line 1

3 Executor, trustee, "care of" name

4a Mailing address (street address) (room, apt., or suite no.)

5a Business address, if different from address in lines 4a and 4b

4b City, state, and ZIP code

5b City, state, and ZIP code

6 County and state where principal business is located

7 Name of principal officer, general partner, grantor, owner, or trustor—SSN required (See instructions.) ▶

8a Type of entity (Check only one box.) (See instructions.)
☐ Estate (SSN of decedent) ______
☐ Trust
☐ Sole Proprietor (SSN) ______
☐ Plan administrator-SSN ______
☐ Partnership
☐ REMIC
☐ Personal service corp.
☐ Other corporation (specify) ______
☐ Farmers' cooperative
☐ State/local government
☐ National guard
☐ Federal government/military
☐ Church or church controlled organization
☐ Other nonprofit organization (specify) ______ (enter GEN if applicable) ______
☐ Other (specify) ▶ ______

8b If a corporation, name the state or foreign country (if applicable) where incorporated ▶ | State | Foreign country

9 Reason for applying (Check only one box.)
☐ Changed type of organization (specify) ▶ ______
☐ Started new business (specify) ▶ ______
☐ Purchased going business
☐ Hired employees
☐ Created a trust (specify) ▶ ______
☐ Created a pension plan (specify type) ▶ ______
☐ Banking purpose (specify) ▶
☐ Other (specify) ▶

10 Date business started or acquired (Mo., day, year) (See instructions.)

11 Enter closing month of accounting year. (See instructions.)

12 First date wages or annuities were paid or will be paid (Mo., day, year). **Note:** *If applicant is a withholding agent, enter date income will first be paid to nonresident alien. (Mo., day, year)* . . . . ▶

13 Enter highest number of employees expected in the next 12 months. **Note:** *If the applicant does not expect to have any employees during the period, enter "0."* . . . . ▶

Nonagricultural	Agricultural	Household

14 Principal activity (See instructions.) ▶

15 Is the principal business activity manufacturing? . . . . ☐ Yes ☐ No
If "Yes," principal product and raw material used ▶

16 To whom are most of the products or services sold? Please check the appropriate box. ☐ Business (wholesale)
☐ Public (retail) ☐ Other (specify) ▶ ☐ N/A

17a Has the applicant ever applied for an identification number for this or any other business? . . . . ☐ Yes ☐ No
Note: *If "Yes," please complete lines 17b and 17c.*

17b If you checked the "Yes" box in line 17a, give applicant's legal name and trade name, if different than name shown on prior application.

Legal name ▶ Trade name ▶

17c Enter approximate date, city, and state where the application was filed and the previous employer identification number if known.

Approximate date when filed (Mo., day, year)	City and state where filed	Previous EIN

Under penalties of perjury, I declare that I have examined this application, and to the best of my knowledge and belief, it is true, correct, and complete

Business telephone number (include area code)

Name and title (Please type or print clearly.) ▶

Signature ▶ Date ▶

Note: *Do not write below this line. For official use only.*

Please leave blank ▶	Geo	Ind.	Class	Size	Reason for applying

For Paperwork Reduction Act Notice, see attached Instructions. Cat. No. 16055N Form **SS-4** (Rev. 12-93)

< **W-2 Wage and tax statement**- As an employer to provide annual wage and tax information to your employee by January 31st of the following year.

a Control number: 22222 | Void ☐ | For Official Use Only ▶

b Employer's identification number: 10- 9876543

c Employer's name, address, and ZIP code:
George M. and Susan A. Adams
718 Poplar Road
Austin, TX 78700

d Employee's social security number: 123-00- 1234

e Employee's name (first, middle initial, last):
Patricia S. Jones
251 Magnolia Way
Austin, TX 78700

f Employee's address and ZIP code

1 Wages, tips, other compensation: 7800.00	2 Federal income tax withheld: 663.00
3 Social security wages: 7800.00	4 Social security tax withheld: 483.60
5 Medicare wages and tips: 7800.00	6 Medicare tax withheld: 113.10
7 Social security tips	8 Allocated tips
9 Advance EIC payment	10 Dependent care benefits
11 Nonqualified plans	12 Benefits included in Box 1
13 See Instrs. for Box 13	14 Other

15 ☐ ☐ ☐ ☐ X ☐ ☐

16 State / Employer's state I.D. No.	17 State wages, tips, etc.	18 State income tax	19 Locality name	20 Local wages, tips, etc.	21 Local income tax
TX / 000-000-10					

Cat. No. 10134D

Department of the Treasury—Internal Revenue Service

W-2 Wage and Tax Statement 1993

Copy A For Social Security Administration

For Paperwork Reduction Act Notice, see separate instructions.

OMB No. 1545-0008

< W-4 Employee's Withholding Allowance Certificate.

The purpose of this form is to allow the employer to withhold the correct amount of Federal Income Tax from an employee's wages.

Form W-4 (1994)

Want More Money In Your Paycheck?
If you expect to be able to take the earned income credit for 1994, you can have part of it added to your take-home pay. For details, get Form W-5 from your employer.

Purpose. Complete Form W-4 so that your employer can withhold the correct amount of Federal income tax from your pay.

Exemption From Withholding. Read line 7 of the certificate below to see if you can claim exempt status. *If exempt, complete line 7; but do not complete lines 5 and 6.* No Federal income tax will be withheld from your pay. Your exemption is good for 1 year only. It expires February 15, 1995.

Note: *You cannot claim exemption from withholding if (1) your income exceeds $600 and includes unearned income (e.g., interest and dividends), and (2) another person can claim you as a dependent on their tax return.*

Basic Instructions. Employees who are not exempt should complete the Personal Allowances Worksheet. Additional worksheets are provided on page 2 for employees to adjust their withholding allowances based on itemized deductions, adjustments to income, or two-earner/two-job situations. Complete all worksheets that apply to your situation. The worksheets will help you figure the number of withholding allowances you are entitled to claim. However, you may claim fewer allowances than this.

Head of Household. Generally, you may claim head of household filing status on your tax return only if you are unmarried and pay more than 50% of the costs of keeping up a home for yourself and your dependent(s) or other qualifying individuals.

Nonwage Income. If you have a large amount of nonwage income, such as interest or dividends, you should consider making estimated tax payments using Form 1040-ES. Otherwise, you may find that you owe additional tax at the end of the year.

Two Earners/Two Jobs. If you have a working spouse or more than one job, figure the total number of allowances you are entitled to claim on all jobs using worksheets from only one Form W-4. This total should be divided among all jobs. Your withholding will usually be most accurate when all allowances are claimed on the W-4 filed for the highest paying job and zero allowances are claimed for the others.

Check Your Withholding. After your W-4 takes effect, you can use **Pub. 919,** Is My Withholding Correct for 1994?, to see how the dollar amount you are having withheld compares to your estimated total annual tax. We recommend you get Pub. 919 especially if you used the Two Earner/Two Job Worksheet and your earnings exceed $150,000 (Single) or $200,000 (Married). Call 1-800-829-3676 to order Pub. 919. Check your telephone directory for the IRS assistance number for further help.

Personal Allowances Worksheet

A Enter "1" for **yourself** if no one else can claim you as a dependent . . . . A ______

B Enter "1" if:
- You are single and have only one job; or
- You are married, have only one job, and your spouse does not work; or
- Your wages from a second job or your spouse's wages (or the total of both) are $1,000 or less.

. . B ______

C Enter "1" for your **spouse.** But, you may choose to enter -0- if you are married and have either a working spouse or more than one job (this may help you avoid having too little tax withheld) . . . . C ______

D Enter number of **dependents** (other than your spouse or yourself) whom you will claim on your tax return . . . . . D ______

E Enter "1" if you will file as **head of household** on your tax return (see conditions under **Head of Household** above) . E ______

F Enter "1" if you have at least $1,500 of **child or dependent care expenses** for which you plan to claim a credit . . F ______

G Add lines A through F and enter total here. **Note:** This amount may be different from the number of exemptions you claim on your return ▶ G ______

For accuracy, do all worksheets that apply.
- If you plan to **itemize or claim adjustments to income** and want to reduce your withholding, **see the** Deductions and Adjustments Worksheet on page 2.
- If you are **single** and have **more than one job** and your combined earnings from all jobs exceed $30,000 OR if you are **married** and have a **working spouse or more than one job,** and the combined earnings from all jobs exceed $50,000, **see** the Two-Earner/Two-Job Worksheet on page 2 if you want to avoid having too little tax withheld.
- If **neither** of the above situations applies, **stop here** and enter the number from line G on line 5 of Form W-4 below.

·················· **Cut here and give the certificate to your employer. Keep the top portion for your records.** ··················

Form **W-4**
Department of the Treasury
Internal Revenue Service

Employee's Withholding Allowance Certificate

▶ For Privacy Act and Paperwork Reduction Act Notice, see reverse.

OMB No. 1545-0010
1994

1 Type or print your first name and middle initial | Last name | 2 Your social security number

Home address (number and street or rural route) | 3 ☐ Single ☐ Married ☐ Married, but withhold at higher Single rate.
Note: If married, but legally separated, or spouse is a nonresident alien, check the Single box.

City or town, state, and ZIP code | 4 If your last name differs from that on your social security card, check here and call 1-800-772-1213 for more information . . . . ▶ ☐

5 Total number of allowances you are claiming (from line G above or from the worksheets on page 2 if they apply) . | 5 |

6 Additional amount, if any, you want withheld from each paycheck . . . . | 6 | $

7 I claim exemption from withholding for 1994 and I certify that I meet **BOTH** of the following conditions for exemption:
- Last year I had a right to a refund of **ALL** Federal income tax withheld because I had **NO** tax liability; **AND**
- This year I expect **a** refund of **ALL** Federal income tax withheld because I expect to have **NO** tax liability.

If you meet both conditions, enter "EXEMPT" here . . . . ▶ | 7 |

Under penalties of perjury, I certify that I am entitled to the number of withholding allowances claimed on this certificate or entitled to claim exempt status.

Employee's signature ▶ **Date ▶** , 19

8 Employer's name and address (Employer: Complete 8 and 10 only if sending to the IRS) | 9 Office code (optional) | 10 Employer identification number

Cat. No. 10220Q

W-5- Earned Income Credit Advance.- This form is used when an employee is eligible to get a portion of earned income credit in advance along with wages.

Form **W-5**
Department of the Treasury
Internal Revenue Service

Earned Income Credit Advance Payment Certificate

1994

Instructions

Changes To Note

If you do not have a qualifying child (defined later), you may be able to claim the earned income credit on your 1994 tax return. But you **cannot** get advance payments of the credit unless you have a qualifying child. Also, the extra credit for a child born during the year and the health insurance credit are no longer allowed.

Purpose

Use Form W-5 if you are eligible to get part of the earned income credit (EIC) in advance with your pay and choose to do so. If you choose not to get advance payments, you can still claim the EIC on your 1994 tax return.

What Is the EIC?

The EIC is a refundable tax credit for certain workers. For 1994, the EIC can be as much as $2,038 if you have one qualifying child; $2,528 if you have more than one qualifying child; $306 if you do not have a qualifying child.

Who Is Eligible To Get Advance EIC Payments?

You are eligible to get advance EIC payments if **all three** of the following apply:

1. You have a qualifying child.

2. You expect that your 1994 earned income and adjusted gross income will each be less than $23,755 (including your spouse's income if you expect to file a joint return).

3. You expect to be able to claim the EIC for 1994. To find out if you may be able to claim the EIC, answer the questions on page 2. If you expect to file **Form 2555**, Foreign Earned Income, or **Form 2555-EZ**, Foreign Earned Income Exclusion, for 1994, you **cannot** claim the EIC.

How Do I Get Advance EIC Payments?

If you are eligible to get advance EIC payments for 1994, you may be able to get up to $102 a month added to your take-home pay. To get advance EIC payments, fill in the Form W-5 at the bottom of this page. Then, detach it and give it to your employer. If you get advance payments, you **must** file a 1994 Form 1040A or Form 1040.

You may have only **one** Form W-5 in effect with a current employer at one time. If you and your spouse are both employed, each of you should file a separate Form W-5.

This Form W-5 expires on December 31, 1994. If you are eligible to get advance EIC payments for 1995, you must file a new Form W-5 next year.

Note: *You may be able to get a larger credit when you file your 1994 return. For details, see* ***Additional Credit*** *on page 2.*

Who Is a Qualifying Child?

Any child who meets **all three** of the following conditions is **a qualifying child**:

1. The child is your son, daughter, adopted child, stepchild, foster child, or a descendant (for example, your grandchild) of your son, daughter, or adopted child.

Note: *An* ***adopted child*** *includes a child placed with you by an authorized placement agency for legal adoption even if the adoption isn't final. A* ***foster child*** *is any child you cared for as your own child.*

2. The child is under age 19 or a full-time student under age 24 at the end of 1994, or is permanently and totally disabled.

3. The child either lives with you in the United States for more than half of 1994 (for all of 1994 if a foster child) OR was born, or died, in 1994 and your home in the United States was the child's home for the entire time he or she was alive.

Note: *Temporary absences such as for school, medical care, or vacation count as time lived with you.*

Married Child.—If the child is married at the end of 1994, the child is a qualifying child only if you may claim the child as your dependent or the **Exception** below applies to you.

Exception. You are the custodial parent and would be able to claim the child as your dependent but the noncustodial parent claims the child as a dependent because—

- You signed **Form 8332**, Release of Claim to Exemption for Child of Divorced or Separated Parents, or a similar statement, agreeing not to claim the child for 1994, or
- You have a pre-1985 divorce decree or separation agreement that allows the noncustodial parent to claim the child and he or she gives at least $600 for the child's support in 1994.

(Continued on page 2)

Give the lower part to your employer; keep the top part for your records.

Detach along this line

Form **W-5**
Department of the Treasury
Internal Revenue Service

Earned Income Credit Advance Payment Certificate

▶ **This certificate expires on December 31, 1994.**

OMB No. 1545-1342

1994

Type or print your full name | **Your social security number**

Note: *If you get advance payments of the earned income credit for 1994, you must file a 1994 Form 1040A or Form 1040. To get advance payments, your filing status must be any status* ***except*** *married filing a separate return and you must have a qualifying child.*

		Yes	No
1	I expect to be able to claim the earned income credit for 1994, I do not have another Form W-5 in effect with any other current employer, and I choose to get advance EIC payments		
2	Do you have a qualifying child?		
3	Are you married?		
4	If you are married, does your spouse have a Form W-5 in effect for 1994 with any employer?		

Under penalties of perjury, I declare that the information I have furnished above is, to the best of my knowledge, true, correct, and complete.

Signature ▶ **Date** ▶

Cat. No. 10227P

 940-EZ and 940- Employer's annual Federal Unemployment Tax (F.U.T.A.) Return.
One of these forms must be filed each year by all employers before January 31st. You make payments called for by using Form 8109 (Federal Tax deposit coupons). You will receive these after you apply for an employer I.D. number.

 942- Employer's Quarterly Tax Return for household employees. You file this form for each quarter of the year, it covers an employee's Social Security, and Medicare taxes, Federal Income Tax, and advanced earned income credit.

 Social Security and Medicare Taxes- Anyone who pays wages of $50.00 or more to an employee in a calendar quarter must pay these taxes. The $50.00 ceiling has been in effect since 1954, and congress has been considering increasing this earnings threshold to as much as $1800.00 per year. Until such legislation may be passed, the $50.00 limit applies for every quarter of a year. You use form 942 to pay Social Security and Medicare Taxes. The total percentage applicable for these taxes is 7.65% of wages paid, 6.2% of which is for Social Security and 1.45% for

Medicare. The combined contributions by the employer and the employee comes to 15.3%. Hence, if you pay your caregiver a salary of $5.00 an hour, or $200.00 a week, here's what you should pay in Social Security, Medicare and other applicable taxes.

Employer Pays:

7.65% S.S. and Medicare: $14.90(subtracted from employee's gross wages)

6.2% Federal Employment Tax: $12.40

Further tax due on the first $7000.00 of an employee's wages is a 2.7% State Employment Tax: $5.40, making your total $32.70 a week if the salary you pay an employee is $200.00.

(The employee's salary after taxes are deducted is $185.10.)

1993 Employee Social Security (6.2%) Tax Deduction Table. (See Circular E for income tax withholding tables.)

Note: *You may use this table to figure how much employee social security tax to deduct from each wage payment. For example, if you pay total wages of $180 during the quarter, the employee tax is $11.16 ($6.20 tax for $100, plus $4.96 for $80 wages). The tax you report on Form 942, line 2, would be $22.32 ($180 × .124 (6.2% employee tax plus 6.2% employer tax)).*

If wage payment is—	The employee tax to be deducted is—	If wage payment is—	The employee tax to be deducted is—	If wage payment is—	The employee tax to be deducted is—	If wage payment is—	The employee tax to be deducted is—	If wage payment is—	The employee tax to be deducted is—
$ 1.00	$ .06	$21.00	$1.30	$41.00	$2.54	$61.00	$3.78	$81.00	$5.02
2.00	.12	22.00	1.36	42.00	2.60	62.00	3.84	82.00	5.08
3.00	.19	23.00	1.43	43.00	2.67	63.00	3.91	83.00	5.15
4.00	.25	24.00	1.49	44.00	2.73	64.00	3.97	84.00	5.21
5.00	.31	25.00	1.55	45.00	2.79	65.00	4.03	85.00	5.27
6.00	.37	26.00	1.61	46.00	2.85	66.00	4.09	86.00	5.33
7.00	.43	27.00	1.67	47.00	2.91	67.00	4.15	87.00	5.39
8.00	.50	28.00	1.74	48.00	2.98	68.00	4.22	88.00	5.46
9.00	.56	29.00	1.80	49.00	3.04	69.00	4.28	89.00	5.52
10.00	.62	30.00	1.86	50.00	3.10	70.00	4.34	90.00	5.58
11.00	.68	31.00	1.92	51.00	3.16	71.00	4.40	91.00	5.64
12.00	.74	32.00	1.98	52.00	3.22	72.00	4.46	92.00	5.70
13.00	.81	33.00	2.05	53.00	3.29	73.00	4.53	93.00	5.77
14.00	.87	34.00	2.11	54.00	3.35	74.00	4.59	94.00	5.83
15.00	.93	35.00	2.17	55.00	3.41	75.00	4.65	95.00	5.89
16.00	.99	36.00	2.23	56.00	3.47	76.00	4.71	96.00	5.95
17.00	1.05	37.00	2.29	57.00	3.53	77.00	4.77	97.00	6.01
18.00	1.12	38.00	2.36	58.00	3.60	78.00	4.84	98.00	6.08
19.00	1.18	39.00	2.42	59.00	3.66	79.00	4.90	99.00	6.14
20.00	1.24	40.00	2.48	60.00	3.72	80.00	4.96	100.00	6.20

Form **942** (Rev. July 1993) Department of the Treasury Internal Revenue Service | 4141

Employer's Quarterly Tax Return for Household Employees

(For Social Security, Medicare, and Withheld Income Taxes) See separate instructions

OMB No 1545-0034

Your name, address, employer identification number, and calendar quarter of return. (If not correct, please change.)

Name: George M. and Susan A. Adams

Date quarter ended: June 30, 1993

Address and ZIP code: 718 Poplar Road, Austin, TX 78700

Employer identification number: - NONE

FOR IRS USE ONLY

If address is different from prior return, check here ▶ ☐

Social security and Medicare taxes are due for each household employee to whom you paid cash wages of $50 or more in the calendar quarter covered by this return. For information on Federal Unemployment (FUTA) Tax, see page 1 of Instructions.

If you will **NOT** need to file Form 942 in the future, check here ▶ ☐

1 Total cash wages subject to social security taxes (see page 2 of Instructions)	1	2400	
2 Social security taxes (multiply line 1 by 12.4% (.124))		2	322 40
3 Total cash wages subject to Medicare taxes (see page 2 of Instructions)	3	2,400	
4 Medicare taxes (multiply line 3 by 2.9% (.029))		4	75 40
5 Federal income tax withheld (if requested by your employee) (see page 2 of Instructions)		5	221 00
6 Total taxes (add lines 2, 4, and 5)		6	618 80
7 Advance earned income credit (EIC) payments ONLY, if any (see page 1 of Instructions)		7	
8 Total taxes due (subtract line 7 from line 6) Pay this amount to the Internal Revenue Service. If no tax is due, write NONE		8	618 80

Send Form 942 and your payment to your **Internal Revenue Service Center (see Where To File on page 2 of Instructions).**

Important: You **MUST** give a Form W-2 to each employee and file Copy A with the **Social Security Administration—see page 3 of Instructions.**

Under the penalties of perjury, I declare that I have examined the return, and to the best of my knowledge and belief, it is true, correct, and complete

Signature of employer ▶ George M. Adams   Date ▶ 7-31-93

Cat No 10250E   Form **942** (Rev 7-93)

Childcare Tax Deductions: Tax deductions for your Federal Income Tax.

 Form 2441- Child and dependent care credit on your Federal Income Tax can be as much as $400.00 for one child and $960.00 for two or more. Your credit decreases as family income increases beyond $10,000. For further information, contact the I.R.S.

Form **2441**

Department of the Treasury
Internal Revenue Service

Child and Dependent Care Expenses

► Attach to Form 1040.

OMB No 1545-0068

1993

21

Name(s) shown on Form 1040 | Your Social Security Number

You need to understand the following terms to complete this form: **Dependent Care Benefits, Earned Income, Qualified Expenses,** and **Qualifying Person(s).** See **Important Terms** in the instructions. Also, if you had a child born in 1993 and line 32 of Form 1040 is less than $23,050, **see A Change to Note** in the instructions.

Part I **Persons or Organizations Who Provided the Care** — **You must complete this part.**
(If you need more space, use the bottom of page 2.)

1 (a) Care providers name	(b) Address (no., street, apt no., city, state, and ZIP code)	(c) Identifying number (SSN or EIN)	(d) Amount paid

2 Add the amounts in column (d) of line 1 2

3 Enter the number of **qualifying persons** cared for in 1993 . . . . ► 3

Did you receive **dependent care benefits?**
- **No** → Complete only Part II below.
- **Yes** → Complete Part III on page 2 now.

Part II **Credit for Child and Dependent Care Expenses**

4 Enter the amount of **qualified expenses** you incurred and paid in 1993. **Do not** enter more than $2,400 for one qualifying person or $4,800 for two or more persons. If you completed Part III, enter the amount from line 25 . . . 4

5 Enter your **earned income** 5

6 If you are filing a joint return, enter **your spouse's** earned income (If student or disabled, see instructions); **all others**, enter the amount from line 5 . . . 6

7 Enter the **smallest** of line 4, 5, or 6 7

8 Enter the amount from Form 1040, line 32 8

9 Enter on line 9 the decimal amount shown below that applies to the amount on line 8 . . . 9

If line 8 is –

Over	But not over	Decimal amount is
$0 –	10,000	.30
10,000 –	12,000	.29
12,000 –	14,000	.28
14,000 –	16,000	.27
16,000 –	18,000	.26
18,000 –	20,000	.25

If line 8 is –

Over	But not over	Decimal amount is
$20,000 –	22,000	.24
22,000 –	24,000	.23
24,000 –	26,000	.22
26,000 –	28,000	.21
28,000 –	No limit	.20

10 Multiply line 7 by the decimal amount on line 9. Enter the result. Then, see the instructions for the amount of credit to enter on Form 1040, line 41 10

Caution: *If you paid $50 or more in a calendar quarter to a person who worked in your home, you must file an employment tax return. Get* **Form 942** *for details.*

D181 **For Paperwork Reduction Act Notice, see separate instructions.** Form **2441** (1993)

Form **2441** (1993) Page **2**

Part III **Dependent Care Benefits** — Complete this part **only** if you received these benefits.

11 Enter the total amount of **dependent care benefits** you received for 1993. This amount should be shown in box 10 of your W-2 form(s). **Do not** include amounts that were reported to you as wages in box 1 of Form(s) W-2	11	
12 Enter the amount forfeited, if any	12	
13 Subtract line 12 from line 11	13	
14 Enter the total amount of **qualified expenses** incurred in 1993 for the care of the qualifying person(s)	14	
15 Enter the **smaller** of line 13 or 14	15	
16 Enter **your earned income**	16	
17 If married filing a joint return, enter **your spouse's** earned income (if student or disabled, see the line 6 instructions); if married filing a separate return, see the instructions for the amount to enter; **all others**, enter the amount from line 16	17	
18 Enter the **smallest** of line 15, 16, or 17	18	
19 **Excluded benefits.** Enter here the **smaller** of the following: • The amount from line 18, or • $5,000 ($2,500 if married filing a separate return **and** you were required to enter your spouse's earned income on line 17).	19	
20 **Taxable benefits**. Subtract line 19 from line 13. Also, include this amount on Form 1040, line 7. On the dotted line next to line 7, write 'DCB'	20	

To claim the child and dependent care credit, complete lines 21 - 25 below, and lines 4 - 10 on page 1 of this form.

21 Enter the amount of qualified expenses you incurred and paid in 1993. **Do not** include on this line any excluded benefits shown on line 19	21	
22 Enter $2,400 ($4,800 if two or more qualifying persons)	22	
23 Enter the amount from line 19	23	
24 Subtract line 23 from line 22. If zero or less, **Stop**. You cannot take the credit. **Exception**. If you paid 1992 expenses in 1993, see the line 10 instructions	24	
25 Enter the **smaller** of line 21 or 24 here **and** on line 4 on page 1 of this form	25	

Form **2441** (1993)

We have discussed above the forms you will need to use for a household employee and your tax responsibilities as an employer. Another matter is what you actually pay to your employee. You can hire a payroll company to keep track of all your tax responsibilities and distribute pay checks to the employee, if you wish and can afford the fee. Another alternative is to purchase a computer program which you can use to calculate Federal Income Taxes, state and local taxes, Social Security taxes, and Federal and State Unemployment taxes. On the next page is an example of a payroll-type check for an employee, set up with the account number and name of your bank on the check. The employee's tax withholdings are calculated and printed for each pay period, and the checks come ready to issue to the employee once the employer endorses them. Mother's Helpmates offers this special service and many others to our clients. If you want more details, contact us at 1-813-681-5183.

COMPANY NAME
ADDRESS
CITY, STATE ZIP

BANK NAME
BRANCH OFFICE
CITY, STATE ZIP
00-6789/0000

11/10/93

PAY TO THE ORDER OF Employee Name $ ********2,742.79

Two Thousand Seven Hundred Forty-Two and 79/100** DOLLARS

Employee Name
Address
City, State Zip

SAMPLE PAYROLL CHECK

VOID

MEMO____________________

COMPANY NAME

Employee Name 11/10/93

Payroll: Gross	YTD Gross Wages	$13269.21	3,750.00
(Payroll-FWH)	YTD Federal Tax	$2142.00	-599.00
(Payroll-SWHCA)	YTD State Tax	$492.42	-121.33
(Payroll-FICA)	YTD Social Sec.	$822.69	-232.50
(Payroll-MCARE)	YTD Medicare	$192.40	-54.38
	Total Hours	:160.00	

1993 Employee Medicare (1.45%) Tax Deduction Table. (See Circular E for income tax withholding tables.)

Note: *You may use this table to figure how much employee Medicare tax to deduct from each wage payment. For example, if you pay total wages of $180 during the quarter, the employee tax is $2.61 ($1.45 tax for $100, plus $1.16 for $80 wages.) The tax you report on Form 942, line 4, would be $5.22 ($180 × .029 (1.45% employee tax plus 1.45% employer tax)).*

If wage payment is—	The employee tax to be deducted is—	If wage payment is—	The employee tax to be deducted is—	If wage payment is—	The employee tax to be deducted is—	If wage payment is—	The employee tax to be deducted is—	If wage payment is—	The employee tax to be deducted is—
$ 1.00	$ .01	$21.00	$ .30	$41.00	$ .59	$61.00	$ .88	$81.00	$1.17
2.00	.03	22.00	.32	42.00	.61	62.00	.90	82.00	1.19
3.00	.04	23.00	.33	43.00	.62	63.00	.91	83.00	1.20
4.00	.06	24.00	.35	44.00	.64	64.00	.93	84.00	1.22
5.00	.07	25.00	.36	45.00	.65	65.00	.94	85.00	1.23
6.00	.09	26.00	.38	46.00	.67	66.00	.96	86.00	1.25
7.00	.10	27.00	.39	47.00	.68	67.00	.97	87.00	1.26
8.00	.12	28.00	.41	48.00	.70	68.00	.99	88.00	1.28
9.00	.13	29.00	.42	49.00	.71	69.00	1.00	89.00	1.29
10.00	.15	30.00	.44	50.00	.73	70.00	1.02	90.00	1.31
11.00	.16	31.00	.45	51.00	.74	71.00	1.03	91.00	1.32
12.00	.17	32.00	.46	52.00	.75	72.00	1.04	92.00	1.33
13.00	.19	33.00	.48	53.00	.77	73.00	1.06	93.00	1.35
14.00	.20	34.00	.49	54.00	.78	74.00	1.07	94.00	1.36
15.00	.22	35.00	.51	55.00	.80	75.00	1.09	95.00	1.38
16.00	.23	36.00	.52	56.00	.81	76.00	1.10	96.00	1.39
17.00	.25	37.00	.54	57.00	.83	77.00	1.12	97.00	1.41
18.00	.26	38.00	.55	58.00	.84	78.00	1.13	98.00	1.42
19.00	.28	39.00	.57	59.00	.86	79.00	1.15	99.00	1.44
20.00	.29	40.00	.58	60.00	.87	80.00	1.16	100.00	1.45

chapter 1

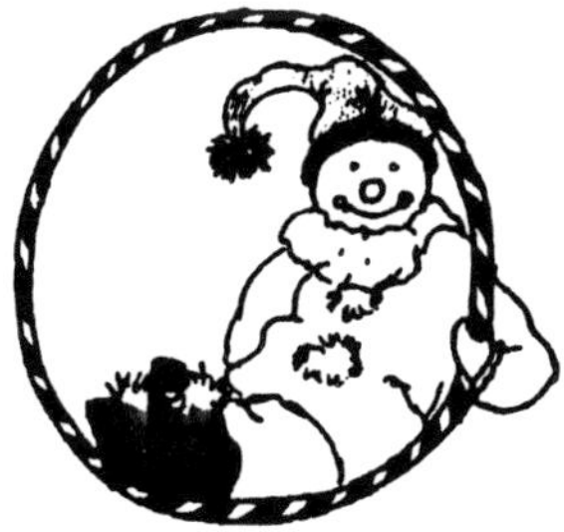

Caws on hiring helpmates

When you become an employer of household help, you will have to comply with many laws. Here are some of them:

Federal Fair Labor Standards Act:
This act applies to domestic service workers. (W.H. Publication 1382)

Employment Eligibility Verification:
You will need to fill out form I-9

Immigration Reform and Control Act of 1986
This says that you should hire only American citizens or those who are authorized to work in the United States.

For more information on these and other laws call 1-202-514-2000 or 1-202-514-4330 1-202-324-5074 at the Justice Department.

Minimum wage is currently $4.25 an hour which is about $4,000 below the poverty level. Most in-home caregivers make a salary of at least $5 - 8 dollars an hour. You should always keep all records on your employees and payments related to them for at least three years. Here are some of the items and information you need to keep:

1.) Name and Social Security number

2) Address and Zip Code

3) Wages paid each week to your employee

4) The total of hours worked each week by all your employees, including overtime.

5) A record of any money paid to your employees for room and board or any money spent on behalf of your live-in or live-out help.

Most states don't require a nanny or household helper to be licensed, but some do. To find out whether there are special laws for nannies in your state, call the Law Enforcement Department. Make sure you have the answer before you hire someone for your home. You can also get such information from your city's or county's licensing department. Save yourself some problems later on by finding out what your local laws are before you hire anyone. Don't risk violating any laws.

chapter 11

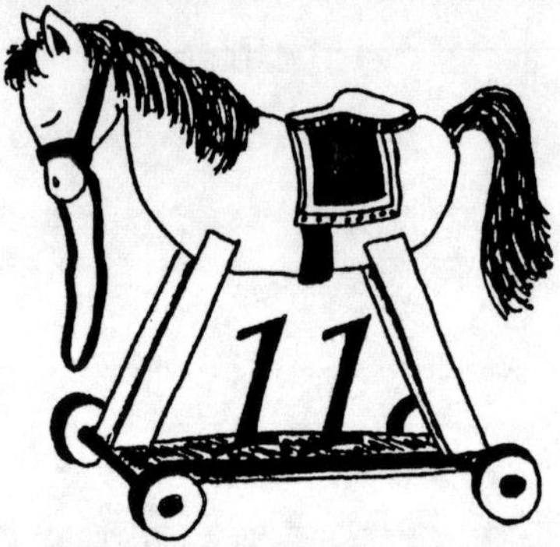

Using a placement agency

When you decide to use an agency, they will apply their experience and expertise to help you in your search for the right employee. Every agency has a network of candidates you alone could not normally, turn up. If you can afford an agency's commission, you will save most of the considerable time it takes to screen prospective caregivers by yourself. Agencies exist on the fees they charge for their services, which will vary from state to state and range from $350.00 to $4,000. The differences in fees are based partly on whether a referral or placement service guarantees placement for 60 days or up to four years. Some agencies will screen the applicants you find on your own for smaller fees. Here are some of the things to do and to look for in choosing an agency:

* Make sure the agency is licensed and inquire how long they have been in business.

* Ask them for references from past clients. However, some agencies may not give out these clients' phone numbers or addresses without first getting their permission.

* Clarify what period the agency's placement

guarantee is good for. Most agencies offer 60-90 day placement guarantees.

* Find out what kind of screening the service provides. Also find out what fees your family will be responsible to pay and what fees the caregiver must pay for. (For example, if the nanny hasn't taken needed training in C.P.R. or first aid, or if they need to re-certify, who will pay for this? Or who will pay for a physical or a drug screen for the nanny or companion if one is requested?

* You might check with the local Better Business Bureau or the Chamber of Commerce to see if the agency is a member in good standing.

* If an agency is a " babysitting" agency, the employees often work for it and the company may be bonded to cover any damages to the client. Be sure to check what the situation is if you are using a baby-sitting or housekeeping agency.

* Ask if the agency has any contract or agreement affecting dealings of the caregiver with any family. You will want to know if there are any binding contracts the agency has that will commit you to pay employee severance pay, insurance, or other costs

you were not aware of. Be sure that you know about all responsibilities placed on you or your employee by any contract between the agency and the employee.

* Find out if the agency offers a payroll program or can refer you to someone who does.

* Make sure the agency provides you copies of references and all available information concerning the employee's background.

* Prepare in advance a written job description for the employee you need which you can show the agency, including the salary you can afford to pay. (See chapters 2 and 3 for examples.)

The costs of using an agency vary according to your precise needs, and will also differ greatly from state to state and city to city. For example you can expect to pay from $450 to $1,000.00 in Tennessee, while in Atlanta you'll pay from $1,000.00 to $4,000.00. An agency that charges $4000.00 will usually give a permanent replacement guarantee, however. Some agencies charge according to your specific need, such as whether you are looking for a live-in or live-out caregiver, for example. Or charges may be based on whether a person needs only a one-day replacement or weekend help. If you hire someone for a few days, you might pay the nanny her fee and then pay the agency for the referral anywhere from $10.00 to $15.00 for each day you use her. Some agencies will screen someone for a small charge without any placement being involved, while others will not do this.

Check around and find out what is offered in your area. If you can't afford the whole placement fee at once, ask whether you can pay in installments. Most agencies want to be paid promptly at usual rates, but if you ask them for help they may be willing to work out a placement fee and terms you would be able to pay.

"Babysitting" agencies charge hourly rates which are a bit higher and the agencies take their fee out of this money. The family may be asked to pay the sitter a couple of dollars a day for car expenses. If you decide to use Au pair services, you will pay the agency a larger placement fee, but the weekly salary for your Au pair will usually be less. Make sure Au pairs have been screened properly by the agency. Learn something about the culture of the country they're from, if they are not American. While the cost may be less, you could get a person whose cultural background doesn't agree with yours.

In general, you get what you pay for, as the old saying goes. So check out all the agencies, find out their costs and what you'll get for your money as far as guarantees and screening are concerned. Then make your choice, and it will probably be a good one.

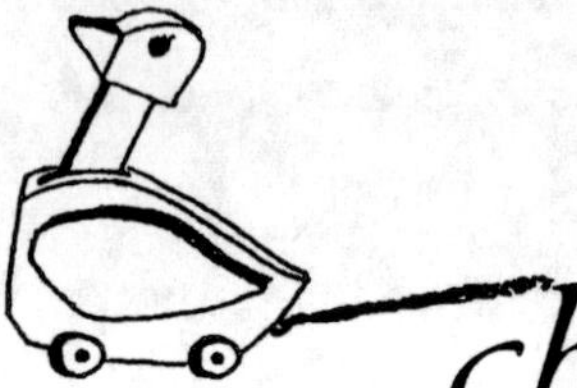

chapter 12

What you need to know about day care and the law.

If you decide a day care center is all you can afford or is best for your child, rather than home care, here are some things to assess and consider in choosing a day care for your child.

* Look at the quality of the day care center's construction and equipment.

* Look at the relationship between the center and the children.

* Review the regulations at the day care. Check to see if they fall within guide lines of the state where you live.

* Check all fire and other safety precautions at the day care center.

* Look around to see if the facility is clean and attractive, for your child will be there most of the day.

* Questions to ask yourself about the day care center or the family day care include the following:

* Are the children happy?

* Is the teacher or provider listening to the children when they talk to her?

* Are the children treated special?

* Are the children encouraged to express themselves?
* What is the ratio of teachers to children at the center?
* Is the schedule of the day structured for the children's benefit?
* What discipline is used at the day care?
* What nutritional value do the daily meals provide for the children's dietary needs?
* Are there restrictions on who is accepted at the day care, such as handicapped children or children on medication for health reasons?
*If they have a pool, is it locked to protect children around the pool area?
* Is any fee charged by the day care if parents are late picking up their child?
* Are the teachers certified in C.P.R? (In some states it is law that all workers must be certified in case of accidents where a child stops breathing .Children are prone to choke easily.)
* Is there time for children to work as a group?
* Does the staff mind if parents drop in during the day

to visit and check on their child?
* Is there a lot of turnover at the daycare?
(This could signal some problem with the center's operations. I hear stories from day care workers all the time about day care centers that are being run poorly by their owners.)
* Do they have any equipment for medical emergencies? (Find out what hospital the center uses in case of accidents or medical problems.)

You can call the YMCA for information on day care centers . They should be able to direct you to day centers, in your area and advise families whose children need after-school care concerning latch-key programs available to them. To check the laws of your state on day care centers contact local offices of the child and welfare department. They will tell you where to get a run-down on state requirements for day care centers.

If the children at a center you visit don't seem happy, check out why. Make sure that the values in the center's program are compatible with yours and that the center will enhance your child's life and promote getting along socially with other children. Children don't like the idea of their parent's just leaving them somewhere. When they are left at a day care, you want to feel they will have fun and learn at the same time. The care you give your children when they are very young will affect their eventual attitudes toward school. You want your children to look forward to going to school, not to dislike it because of past bad experience at a day care.

Day cares should provide stimulation for children and encourage them to play together, Its activities should allow the children to experiment with new materials and try new experiences. There should be a time each day for outside play. The toys at the center should challenge a child's learning skills, whether puzzles, books, or building materials. There should be opportunities for trips away from the center for exposure to new people and experiences. The teacher or caregiver might sometimes take the children for walks or to a museum or library. When the center provides such activities for children, it helps them develop social skills and discover where they stand in the world around them.

Here are some laws on day care centers to look

for in the state where you live. Most states' laws cover many of the same areas as Florida 's day care laws, which are as follows:

(1) Family day care homes may be licensed by the state if they are currently licensed by one of its counties. Family day cares must register annually with the state the home's name and address, the name of its operator, the number of children it provides care for, and the availability of emergency equipment.

(2) This information is included in a directory published annually by the state's Department of Licensing.

(3) Child care personnel in family day care homes shall be subject to applicable screening provisions of ss. 402.305. (1)(a) and 402.3055.

(4) Operators of family day care homes must take an approved three hour introductory course in child care.

(5) Family day care home operators may avail themselves of the supporting services of the Department of Licensing.

(6) This Department will prepare a brochure on family day care for distribution by itself and local licensing departments, including:

(a) A brief description of the requirements for day care registration, training, fingerprinting and screening.
(b) A listing of counties that require family home day cares and information concerning the licensing.
(c) A statement about family day care home's compliance with state law and local requirements can be obtained by telephoning the Department of Licensing.
(d) The state wide telephone number of the Florida Abuse Registry, plus reports of suspected and actual abuses by day cares.
(e) Any other information relating to competent child care which the Department or local licensing agencies deem helpful to the public.
(7) The Department also must prepare an annual evaluation of the registration and licensure system for family day care homes which includes, at a minimum, the following:
(a) The number of family day care homes registered.
(b) The number of children taken care of by home day care.
(c) The number of complaints concerning family home day care.

(d.) The training activities being utilized by the day cares, according to local training requirements.

(8) In order to inform the public of the state requirements for registration of family day care homes and other requirements for such homes to operate legally, the state shall institute a media campaign via flyers, television, radio or newspaper advertisements, etc.

Licensing standards for child care facilities are as follows:

(1) Personnel- Minimum standards for child care personnel, whether employees or volunteers, to include minimum age requirements, minimum staff training requirements for identification and reporting of child abuse and neglect, periodic health examinations, minimum levels of training in first aid, and ratios of personnel to children.

(2) Physical facilities- Minimum standards for building and conditions, indoor play space, outdoor play space, napping space, bathroom facilities, food preparation facilities, outdoor equipment and indoor equipment.

(3) Sanitation and safety.-Minimum standards for

sanitary and safety conditions, first aid treatment, and emergency procedures.

(4) Nutritional practices.- Minimum standards for the provision of meals or snacks of a quality and quantity to assure that the nutritional needs of children are met.

(5) Admissions and record keeping.- Requirements for pre-admission and periodic health examinations, requirements for immunizations, requirements for maintaining emergency information and health records for all children. Any child may be exempted from medical or physical examination, or medical or surgical treatment, upon written request of the child's parent or guardian who objects to the examination or treatment. However, no laws, rules and regulations relating to contagious or communicable diseases and sanitary matters shall be violated.

(6) Transportation safety.- Requirements for child restraints or seat belts in vehicles used by child care facilities to transport children, requirements for annual inspections of the vehicles and limitations on facilities to transport children, requirements for annual inspections of the vehicles and limitations on the number of children in the vehicles.

(7) Access.- Minimum standards that provide for reasonable access to the child care facility by the custodial parent or guardian during the time the child is in care.

(8) Child Discipline.- Minimum standards for child discipline practices to ensure that age-appropriate, constructive disciplinary practices are used for children in care. Such standards shall include at least the following minimum requirements:

(a) Children shall not be subject to discipline which is severe, humiliating, or frightening.

(b) Discipline shall not be associated with food, rest, or toileting.

(c) Spanking or any other form of physical punishment is prohibited.

(9) Plan of activities.- Minimum standards to ensure that each child care facility implements a written plan for daily provision of varied activities and active and quiet play opportunities appropriate to the age of the children.

Here is a check list to use when interviewing the day care you are considering for your child.

NAME OF THE CENTER____________DATE___
ADDRESS OF THE DAY CARE OR FAMILY HOME DAY CARE:____
INFORMATION ON THE PROGRAMS THEY PROVIDE AT THE CENTER____
ARE THE PROGRAMS THEY PROVIDE LICENSED?
YES [] NO[]
ARE THE HOURS THEY ARE OPENED ACCEPTABLE AND FLEXIBLE FOR YOUR JOB SCHEDULE?
YES [] NO []
IS THE COST OF THE CENTER AFFORDABLE FOR YOUR FAMILY?
YES [] NO []
HOW WOULD YOU GRADE THE ATMOSPHERE OF THE DAY CARE ? GOOD [] FAIR []
IS THE DAY CARE SAFE AND WELL MAINTAINED?
YES []NO []
IS THE DAY CARE CHEERFUL?
YES []NO []
ARE THE TOYS SAFE AND CLEAN ?
YES [] NO []
HAS THE DAY CARE ENOUGH LIGHT AND VENTILATION?
YES [] NO []
DO THEY HAVE FIRE EXTINGUISHERS AND SMOKE DETECTORS?
YES [] NO []
DO THEY HAVE MEDICINES AND HOUSEHOLD PRODUCTS LOCKED AWAY FOR SAFETY FROM THE CHILDREN?
YES [] NO []

LOOK AT THE CAREGIVERS AND ASK YOURSELF THESE QUESTIONS: DOES THE SUPERVISOR SEEM TO ENJOY THE CHILDREN AT THE CENTER OR HOME?
YES [] N0 []
THE WORKERS RESPOND QUICKLY TO THE CHILDREN'S NEED?
YES [] NO []
DOES THE CAREGIVERS PLAY OR INTERACT WITH THE CHILDREN?
YES [] NO []
ARE THE CHILDREN HANDLED GENTLY?
YES [] NO []
ARE THE ACTIVITIES AT THE DAY CARE VARIED AND AGE APPROPRIATE?
YES [] NO []
DO THE CHILDREN PLAY OUTDOORS?
YES [] NO[]
IS THERE A CLEAR SCHEDULE FOR MEALS , NAP, PLAY TIME ?
YES [] NO []
CAN THE PARENTS VISIT THE CENTER?
YES [] NO[]
ARE THEY ENCOURAGED TO MEET WITH THE CAREGIVER REGULARLY?
YES [] NO[]
WHAT IS YOUR GENERAL REACTION TO THE DAY CARE OR FAMILY?
YES [] NO[]
HOME DAYCARE?
YES [] NO[]

Make sure you are comfortable with every aspect of the day care you are considering for your child. Remember your child or children will be there most of the day and you want them to be happy, comfortable, and safe. Always check the state authorities where you live to familiarize yourself with any laws concerning day care in your area. The laws we have discussed here are those of the state of Florida, but most laws concerning day care are similar in other states. Make sure the day care center you are interested in abides by all the state's laws for the safety of your child or children.

LIST OF STATE STATUTES FOR DAY CARE AND OTHER CHILD CARE ORGANIZATIONS IN THE UNITED STATES :

For a full description of these laws and statutes contact: The National Crime Information Center

10th and Pennsylvania Avenue,

N.W. Washington, DC 20535

Alabama- Statute H. 941 ACT 85-537 pertains to public and private day care and child care facilities and personnel. This law also includes child in-home care.

Alaska- Statute AS 12. 62.035 pertains to employment of those having supervisory or disciplinary power over minors including day-care centers and babysitters.

Arizona- ARS 36-882 and 36-83.02 pertains to applicants for daycare center licenses and employees of day care centers. ARS 36-897.01 and 36- 897.03 pertains to day care applicants for day care group home certification and child care personnel of day care group homes.

Arkansas- ARS 20-78-602 pertains to child care facilities, owners, operators and employables 20-78-602.

California- Sec. 1. 3, Sect. 1522 H. & S C pertains to child care and home finding agencies, adult care homes and facilities. Sections 1597.81 and 1597.82 of the California Assembly Bill No. 3961 pertains to child care providers.

Colorado-CRS 26-6-107 pertains to applicants for license to

operate the following: Family care home, residential child care facility, child placement agency, and child care centers.

Connecticut- CGSA 54-142K pertains to care or treatment of children.

Delaware- 31 DC section 309 pertains to child care personnel.

Florida- F. S. Chapter 394 pertains to child care facility, family day care home, residential child care agency, child placing agency. F.S. 394 pertains to day care or residential facility caretakers providing treatment to retarded or disabled children or adults.

Georgia- OCGA Sec. 31-7-254 pertains to licensing of directors and employees of personal care homes. OCGS Sec. 49-5-64 pertains to licensing of directors and employees of child care centers.

Hawaii- HRS CH. 346, ACT 208 of 1985 pertains to the operators and employees of child-care institutions , child-placing organizations and foster boarding homes.

Idaho- Section 67-2931 Idaho code, permits local government non-law enforcement agencies to require fingerprinting by rule, regulation, or ordinance applicable to employment and licensing. Sec. 39-1101 through 39-1117 pertains to child day care.(There are different statutes in different counties in Idaho so you should contact your county authorities for what may apply to you.)

Illinois- ISC, Chap. 122 , Sec. 10-21 9 & 34-18.5 pertains to child care licensing.

Maryland- Family Law Article, 5-551 (c) (iii) , pertains to registration of providers at family day care homes for children. For background check re:children, See ACM 5-560 through 5-551. Includes employers, employees and adult volunteers providing care supervising children in the following settings child care centers, family day-care home, child care homes, child care institutions, or homes of adult relatives where a child is placed by the MDSS.

Minnesota- MS 2451. 04 Subd. 3 (a) & (b) (3) pertains to human services applicant, including employees, contractors, or volunteers who work in applicable child care. Section 299C. 62 MS pertains to child service providers and their employees.

Missouri- RSMO Section 43.543 pertains to applicants for license/employment with state agencies which provide care or treatment or exercise supervision over minors.

Nevada- NRS 432A.175 pertains to licensing and employment of applicants and residents of child care facilities. NRS 179A.210 pertains to employees and volunteers working with children.

New Jersey-.S.B. 1721; NJSA 30: 5B -26 pertains to child care of school children before and after school.

New Mexico- NMSB 247 pertains to operators , staff, and employees of child care facilities.

North Carolina- NCGS 110-90.1 through 110-91 pertains to staff of child day care plans and child day care facilities

North Dakota- Statute 50-11. 106.02 NDCC pertains to child care providers.

Ohio- ORC 109.572 pertains to background checking of

applicants responsible for the care, custody, or control of a child. ORC 2151.86 pertains to out-of-home child care and ORC 5104.012 and 5104.013 to child day care centers.

Oregon- ORS 181.537 pertains to applicants relating to the care or treatment of children.

Pennsylvania- Child Protective Services Law, ACT 33 of 1985, Sec. 23.1 pertains to child care services applicants, family day care providers and other child-care facilities or programs

Rhode Island- RIGL 40-13.2-40-13-4 pertains to licensing and employment of childcare personnel.

South Carolina- Sections 26-6-14.3 through 26.6-14.5 SDCL pertains to adults or volunteers who provide care or supervision to children and adults.

Tennessee- HB 472 pertains to adults or volunteers who provide care or supervision to children and adults.

Texas- Department of Protective and Regulatory Services S411.087 and 411.114 GC pertains to owners, employees and applicants of childcare facilities, home health care facilities, in-home respite care of children, and applicants for license, registration, or certification in connection with child care facilities.

Washington- Statute 28A. 400 RCW pertains to employees and contractors who have unsupervised access to children.

West Virginia- Statue WVC 49-2 B-8 pertains to child care agencies and applicants.

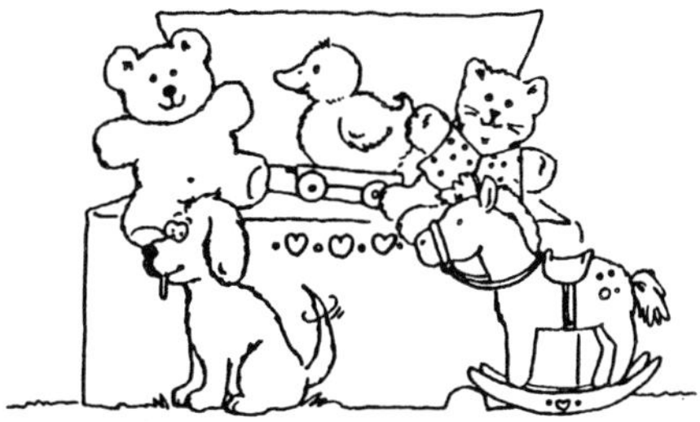

Appendix A

Listing of nanny training schools in the United States.

(Mother's Helpmates can't guarantee the information is accurate or that the schools, agencies, services, etc. listed provide quality services or training. Please check with the schools, agencies, services, etc. to verify the information listed.)

Nanny Schools in the United States

American Nanny College
4650 Arrow High Suite A-10, Montclair, CA 91763
909-624-7711

American Nanny College
P.O Box 790, Claremont, CA 95825
1-714-624-7711 800-462-7711
30 hrs of work with children.
cost $4,795

Care -4-Kids ,INC.
1207 Glance Ave, Highland Park,IL 60035-4007
1-708- 433-4737
Monthly 48 hrs total
Monthly 3 hour seminars offered continuously.
cost $1,200

Caregivers Training School
155 Chestnut St., West Springfield, MA 01103
413-737-2525

Appendix A: Listing of nanny schools in the United States.

Carl Sandburg College
2232 S. Lake Storey, Galesgurg, IL 61401
309-433-4738
2 Semesters 32 hr credit
cost $1,500

Central Community College
East Highway 6, Hastings , NE 68901
402-463-9811

Central Community College
613 North Washington St., Lexington, NE 68850
308-324-5936

Central Community College
512 W. 11 th St., Kearney, NE 68847
308-237-2379

Colorado Nanny Academy
17800 Road, Fort Morgan,CO. 80701
303-867- 6608
2 semester cost $1900.00 120 hours

Community College of Allegheny County
North Campus, 8701 Perry Highway, Pittsburgh, PA. 15237
412-369-3624
9 months cost -$1,394
18 months hrs.- Assoc. 9 months -cost $2,787

Appendix A: Listing of nanny schools in the United States.

Delta College
University Center, Michigan 48710
1-517-686-9543

Demarge College Inc.
3608 N.W. 58th Street, Oklahoma City, OK. 73112
405-947-1534
19 weeks- cost $3,995 certificate

English Nanny & Governess School
30 South Frankilin ,Chargrin Falls, OH.44022
800-733-1984- fax
cost $3000.00 3 month Course

Independent Community College
P.O. Box 708, Independence , KS.
316- 331-4100
350 hrs 4 semester cost
$25.00 per credit. $73.00 out of state.

Metro Tech. Vo Tech.
Dist. No. 22 3901 N. Maritin Luther, Oklahoma City , OK. 73111
405-424-8324

Metro Tech Vocnl Techl Centers
5600 S .Macarthur Blvd. Oklahoma, OK
405-424-8324

Montana Nannies ,Inc
101 11th Ave. S., Shelby, MT 59474
406-434-2502
cost $1445 75 hrs by correspondence source. 100 hrs work

Moraine Park Technical College
235 North National Ave, Fond Du Lac, WI
414-922 8611
800- 221L16430
1,030 hours one year $1700. cost

Moraine Technical College
700 Goluld St., Beaver Dam, WI 53916
414-887-1101

Moraine Technical College
742 Greentree Mall, Berlin, WI 54923
414-361-3601

Morgan Community College
17800 County Road 20, Fort Morgan, CO 80701
303-867-3081

Muffy Vrana & Company
3260 Van Dorn, Lincoln, NE 68502
402-488-0316
Home Study Course Fee Negotiable

Appendix A: Listing of nanny schools in the United States.

Murray State College
Rt.1, Box 84, Tishominga, OK 73460
405- 371-2371
384 class hours cost $29.30 credit hour. 384 work

Nannies of America
4190 Telegraph, Suite 3300, Bloomfield, MI 48302
313-540-4960

Nannies of Kentucky
4300 W Highway 146, Crestwood, KY 40014
502-222-7690

Nanny's & Granny's
6440 W. Coley, Las Vegas, NV 9102
702-364-5901
440 16 weeks $2000

Nanny's & Granny's
Neighborhood Nannies 205, Haddonfield, N.J. 08033
609-795-5833
260 hours -40 hours - cost $1,220

Nanny's & Granny's
3790 Redwood St., Las Vegas, NV 89103
702-362-9255

Appendix A: Listing of nanny schools in the United States.

Nanny's & Granny's
South Highland Dr., Las Vegas, NV 89103
702-368-7741

New World Nannies Inc.
8706 Melwood Lane, Richmond, VA 23229
804-282-6128
160 hours 50 hr work cost $900.00

NMSU Dona Ana Branch Community College
Box 30001, Dept. .3 D.A.,   Las Cruces, NM 88003
505-527-7515
300 hrs 200 hours work $388.00

Northeastern Oklahoma A.&M. College
Box 3894, Miami ,OK 74354
918-542-8441
544 hrs cost $3,300

Quapaw Technical Institute
200 Mid -American Blvd., Hot Springs, AR 71913
501- 767-9314
480 hrs 480 work cost $240.00 per semester

Red Wing Technical College
5354 Moundsview Dr., Red Wing, MN 55066
800- 657-4849
900 hours 675 work   cost $2,182.00

Appendix A: Listing of nanny schools in the United States.

Southeast Community College
Lincoln, NE 68520
402-437-2455
581 hours- 491 work - cost year $1550

Sullivan County Community College
Early Childhood Programs,
Box 4002 Loch, Sheldrake, NY.12759
914-434-5750
39 hrs certificate- 66 hrs Associate cost is 1 yr. $5,200-
2 years Certificate $10.00

Vermont School for Nannies
207-232 Skitchewaug Trail, Springfield, VT 05156
802- 885-3556
240 hrs- 300 work cost 3 month $2,100

University of New Mexico
Los Almos 400 University Dr.,, Los, Alamos, NM 87544
505-662-5919
200 hrs 100 hours work cost $450.00/$5.50

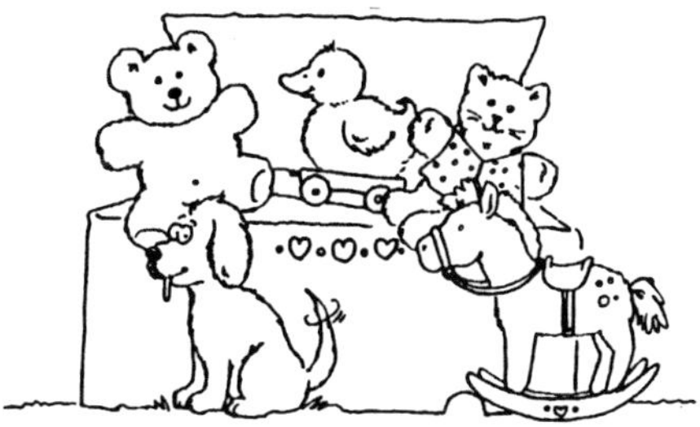

Appendix B
Cisting of nanny, companion,sitter, caregiver, and house sitting agencies and services in the United State.

(Mother's Helpmates can't guarantee the information is accurate or that the schools, agencies, services, etc. listed provide quality services or training. Please check with the schools, agencies, services, etc. to verify the information listed.)

Nanny, Companion, Sitter, Caregiver, and House Sitting Agencies and Services in the United States.

A Caring Nanny
3314 Henderson, Blvd. Suite 100, Tampa, Fl
813-870-6269

A Choice Nanny
681 Lexington Ave., New York, NY 10022
212-246-5437

A Choice Nanny
11 Continental Drive , 108, Newark DE 19713
302-292-0626
Fee $150

A Choice Nanny
7232 Sand Lake Rd. Suite 305, Orlando, FL 32819
407-876-1666
$100 & $1,200

A Choice Nanny
1413 S. Howard Ave. Suite 201, Tampa, FL 33606
813-254-8687
$100 & $1,200

A Choice Nanny
8827 Columbia 100 Parkway ,Suite 1 A, Columbia, M.D 21045
410-730-2229
$100, $400 to $1,200

A Choice Nanny
7300 York Rd, Suite 101, Towson, MD 21204
410-823-8687
$100 & $1,000- $1,200

A Choice Nanny
248 Columbia Turnpike, Florham Park, NJ 07728
908-780-3037

A Choice Nanny
2530 Riva RD., Annapolis, MD 21401
410-730-2356

A Choice Nanny
Rt. 9 Barkalow Ave., Freehold, NJ 07728
908-780-3037
Registration $100

A Choice Nanny
27 Mountain Blvd. Suite 9 B., Warren, NJ 07059
908-754-9090

Appendix B: Listing of nanny agencies and other services in the US.

A Choice Nanny
637 Wyckoff Ave., Wyckoff Ave, NJ 07481
201-891-1722
Fee $125 to $1,300

A Choice Nanny
130 57th St. Suite 4 E., New York, NY 10019
212-246- KIDS

A Choice Nanny
1911 North Fort Myer Dr. No.. 307, Rossyn, VA 22209
800-296-2261
$125 & $600to $1,200

A Choice Nanny
8230 Leesburg Pike, Vienna, VA 22182
703-827-2716
Registration .$25 To $125 $900 to $!,400

A Friend of the Family
895 Mt. Vernon Highway, Atlanta, GA 30327
404-255-2848
Fee $750 to $2,300

A Nanny World Ltd.
6001 Staples Mill Rd., Richmond, VA 23228
804-262-1900

A New England Nanny, Ltd.
2 Strawtown. Rd., West Nyack, NY 10994
914-353-4778
Registration .$75 & $475 to $975

Adele Poston /Park Ave./Bonfield Domestic Agencies
16th East 79th St., New York, NY 10021
212-879-7474
30% of nanny's salary

American Nanny Plan
700 Locust Suite 104, Des Moines, IA 50309
515-245-4279
Registration $25 & $75 Fee $500

American Nanny Plan
4650 Arrow Hwy, No. A-10, Montclair, CA 91763
909-624-7711
Registration $25 10% of nanny's annual salary.

Apple Pie
551 Valley Rd. Suite 188 Upper, Montclair, NJ 07043
201-589-3807 800- 598-3807
Registration $25 & $1,500

Appendix B: Listing of nanny agencies and other services in the US.

Ascot Nannies of Greater New York Inc.
28 Lafayette PL., Greenwich, CT 06830
203-629-2200
Fee $1,400

Ashford Nannies
P.O. Box 22529, Kanas City, MO 64113

At Your Service Agency
120 Country Rd., Tenafly, NJ 07670
202-894-5339
$1,400 or 4 weeks of nanny's salary

Au Pair Extraordiaire
Granda Hills, CA 91344
818-366-4420

Au Pair Extraordiaire
6105 West 6th St., Los Angeles , CA 90048
818-831-9032
Registration $150 Fee is one month of nanny's salary

Au Pair Homestay, U.S.A.
1015 15th St. N.W. Suite 750, Washington , DC 20005
202-408-5380
Registration $75 Fee not listed.

Au Pair Home Stay USA
San Jose, CA 95125
408-264-0677

Au Pair In America
Boulder, CO 80302
303-443-5206

Au Pair In America
Concord, MA 01742
508-369-2348

Au Pair Programme USA
36 South State ST. Suite 3000, Salt Lake City, UT 84111
801-943-7788
Registration $175 Fee $3,175

Au Pair Professionals of Boston
135 Selwyn Rd., Newton, MA 02161
617-527-0114
Fee $1,400

Aunt Ann's Agency
760 Market No. 539, San Francisco, CA 94102
415-421-8442
Fee 75 % of nanny's salary

Appendix B: Listing of nanny agencies and other services in the US.

Baby Nurses LTD

11941 Wilshire BLVD No. -26, Los, Angeles, CA 90025

310-477- 3812

Baby Sitters Agency Bureau & Registry

103 Windy Pl, Brandon, FL 33511

813-681-2002

$5.50 an hour

Minimum of 4 hours & 3 dollars transportation charge.

Baby Sitters Agency Bureau

Santa Monica Marina, Del Rey, CA 91030

310-306-5437

Baby Sitters DLS Inc. EMP Service

2703 Fondren Dr. NO. -130, Dallas, TX 77089

Baby Sitting Service

Sererna Park, MD 21146

410-544-6499

Baby Sitting Placement Service

1550 Worchester Rd,.Framingham, MA 017015

508-872-8428

Baby Sitting Service

St. Petersburg, FL

813-525-1094

Baby Sitting Register
210 Chestnut St., Market, OH 45750
614-373-1410

B. & G. Regal Domestics Inc. P.o
Box 34557, Bethesda , MD 20817
301-469-6817
9 % to 12 % of nanny's salary

Baby Buddies Agency Inc.
144. S. Beverly Dr., Beverly Hills, CA 90212
310-273-2330
Fee 10 % of nanny's salary

Bay Area Second Mom
644 Towle Pl., Palo Alto, CA 94306
415-858-2469
Fee $1,200

Be In Our Care
31 La Mesa Ln., Walnut Creek, CA 94589
510-933-2273
Fee one month of nanny's salary

Be My Nanny
P.O.Box 8777, Madison, WA 53708
608-277-8282

Appendix B: Listing of nanny agencies and other services in the US.

Beacon Hill Nannies Inc.

440 Commercial St., Boston, MA 02109

617-227-5592

$125 to $375

Best Nanny Employment Agency Inc.

1496 Registertown Rd. Suite 108, Baltimore, MD 21208-

410-486-2135

Registration $100 Fee $1,200

Birmingham Home Services Inc.

Office Park Circle , Bldg. 16, Suite 4, Birmingham, Al 35223

205-871-2032

Registration $100 $200 to $600

British Nanny Service

4595 Chestnut Ridge Rd. No. -1, Amhearst, NY 14228

716-877-0726

Buckingham, Nannies

14542 Venture Blvd. Suite 2008, Sheman Oaks, CA 91423

818-784-6504

Capable Care of Maryland Inc.

5110 Ridgefield Rd. no. 212, Bethesda, MD 20816

301-718-3700

Registration $50 Fee Not listed

Capable Care Of Pa. Inc.
1 Executive Blvd., Blue Bell, PA
215-941-0336
Registration $50 Fee Not listed

Capable Care of Va. Inc.
8230 Leesburg Pike, Suite Vienna, VA 22182
703-556-4495
Registration $50 Fee $1,100

Care For Kids Inc.
P.B. Box 27, Rowayton, CT 06853
203-838-7356
Fee $1,500

Care For Kids Inc.
1207 Glencoe Ave, Highland Park, IL 60035
708-433-4737
10% of nanny salary or $10.00 a day for temporary

Care Finders Inc.
1 Grove St. Suite 112, Pittsford, NY 14534
716-381-4840
Fee $975 to $1,600

Appendix B: Listing of nanny agencies and other services in the US.

Care Givers Placement
4004 SW Kelly Ave., Portland, OR 97201
503-245-4814
Fee $750

CareQuest Inc.
2 Broad St. Third Floor, Red Bank, NJ 07701
908-842-1660
Registration $50 Fee $850

Caring Nannies of San Antonio
P.O. Box 780063, San Antonio, TX 78278
210-666-2669
Registration $100 Fee $850

Carriage Trade Nannies
3239 Juniper Lane Falls, Church, VA 22044-1610
703-534-1151

Cass & Co. Inc.
1 Richmond Square, Providence, RI 02906
401-792-0521
$850 to $1,500

Chapel Hill Nannies ,Inc.
Box 9243, Chapel Hill, NC 27515
919-942-9915
Registration $50 Fee $950

Child Care of Dupage ,Inc.
27 W 170 Sycamore, Winfield, IL 60190
708-665-7007
Fee $750 to $900

Child Care Placement Service ,Inc.
149 Buckminster Rd., Brookline, MA 02146
617-566-3657
Fee. $1,600 to one month of nanny's salary

Child Care Professionals Inc.
6576 Maderira Hills Dr., Cincinnati, OH 45243
513-561-4810
Registration $75 Fee one month of nanny's salary or $900

Child Care Service Of Wisconsin
P.O. Box 26943, Wauwatosa,WI 53226
414-782-4276
Registration $50 Fee $800

Childcrest
36 South State, Suite 3000, Salt Lake City, UT 84111
801-943-5527
Fee $1,285

Appendix B: Listing of nanny agencies and other services in the US.

Childminders Inc.
4350 Oakton, Suite 204, Skokie, IL 60076
708- 673-8998
Fee $900

Classics Nannies
264 "H" St.,Blaine, WA 98230
800-663-6128
Fee $800.00

Companions & Sitters
115 Sally Ln., Madison, AL 35758
205-772-8246

Companion For Children Inc.
12 Main St. S., Minot, ND 58701

Companions Nurses & Nannies
2 Bow Cir., Hilton Head Island, SC 29928
803-785-3600

Companion Sitter Services
RR 2, Winterville, NC 27909
919-338-5768

Companions Sitter Service
Headline ,AL 36345
205-693-5525

Connecticut Nanny Inc.
P.O.Box 931, Litchfield, CT 06759
203-567-3813
Placement $950.00

C & I Nanny Professionals
245 East 6th Street Suite 703, St. Paul, MN 55101
612-221-0587
Registration $100 Placement $950

Dependable Nursing & Family Care Inc.
101 W. Robert E. Lee ,Suite 201, New Orleans, LA 70124
504- 282-2200, 800-862-5806
Fee$ 1,200

Dial A Mom Inc.
2659 Towngate Rd. No. 108, Westlake Village, CA 91361
805-496-2264
Fee 70% of nanny's first month salary.

Dial A Sitter, Inc.
1665 Spring Ridge Cr., Wintergarden, FL 34787
800-472-7121, 407-877-6388
Registration $60 Fee $240

Appendix B: Listing of nanny agencies and other services in the US.

Distinctive Domestic Inc.

3000 E. Sunrise Blvd. No. 5 E., Fort Lauderdale, FL 33304

305-564-8229

Registration 150 $250 to $750

EF Au Pair

One Memorial Drive, Cambridge, MA 02142

617-252-6145, 800-333-6056

Registration $175 Fee $3,190

Elderly Care Help Organization

211 Sherwood Dr., Zelienople, PA 16063

412-772-0051

Elderly Care Referral Service

Tucson, AZ 85718

602-529-0553

Elderly Care Calling Service

310 W River Dr., Davenport, IA 52801

319-324-2007

Elderly Care Coordination Services

610 Indiana Ave, Saint Mary's ,OH 45885

419-394-3608

Elderly Day Care Center
225 E High St., Lima, OH 45806
419-228-2688

Elderly Care
28009 118th Ave SE, Kent, WA 98031
206-631-8959

English Nannies & Governess Ltd
24301 Bryden Rd., Beachwood, OH 44122
216-247-0602
Registration $125 Fee $1,700

Exclusive-ly Nannies
P.O. Box 1068, West Brook, ME 04092
207-871-8227
Registration $15 Fee $600

Fairchild Nanny Service
10061 Talbert Ave. Suite 202, Fountain Valley, CA 92708
714-965-5642
Fee one month of nanny's salary

Family Care Necessities
57 Union Place, Suite 212, Summit, NJ 07901
908-273-2299
800-care-4-co

Appendix B: Listing of nanny agencies and other services in the US.

Family Extensions , Inc.
244 Elm St., New Canaan ,CT 06840
203-966-9737
Registration $25 Fee 12% of annual gross salary of nanny

Friend of the Family of Kansas City
12414 Summit St, .Kansas City, MO 64145
406-542-0241
Registration $400 to $450

Heartland Nannies & Companies to Elderly
5500 Grant Creek Rd, Missoula, MT 59802
406-542-0241
Registration $135 Fee $1,200

Heartland Nannies Regularly
P.O. Box 1582, North Platte, NE 69101
308-532-7504, 800-336-9783
Registration $50 $1,000

Heaven Sent Nannies
Lakeview Condos ,No. 293, Enfield, NH 03748
603-632-4108
Registration $75 Fee 4750 to $9.95

Help!
15 Bridge Rd, Weston, CT 06883
203-226-3456, 203-226-HELP
Fee One month's salary $1400 min.

Help Mates Unlimited
3 Terrace Dr., Bethel, CT 06801
1-800-live-ins, 203-274-7511
Registration $125 Fee $999

Helpers West
P.O. box 944, Highland, UT 84003
801-756-8700
Fee $1,500

Helping Hand
5656 West College, Phoenix, AZ 85031
602-846-5908

Helping Hands (Childcare Connexion)
P.O.Box 237, Greenwich, CT 06836
800-544-nani
Fee $1,850

Here's Help ! Inc.
3251 Sacramento St., San Francisco, CA 94115
415-563-0242
75% of the nanny's salary

Appendix B: Listing of nanny agencies and other services in the US.

Home Buddies
1000 Airport Rd. Suite 11, Huntsville, AL 35802
205-882-1299
Fee $300

Home Management Services ,Inc.
8070 Beechmont Ave, Cincinnati ,OH 45255
513-474-5800
Registration $50 $300

House Sitters
1045 Terrace Dr., Saint Louis, MO 63117
614-373-1410

House Sitters
8619 Shauna Oaks Cir N, Jacksonville, FL 32211
904-745-5252

House Sitters International
Hudson, OH 44236
216-650-6428

I Love My Nanny
1072 S. Saratoga-s Vale Rd. Suite B203, San Jose, CA 95129
408-99-Nanny
Fee varies

I Love My Nanny
Palo Alto, CA 94301
415-326-0216

Indy Nannies Plus, Inc.
7240 Shadeland Sta. Way, Suite 114, Indianapolis, IN 46256
Fee $995

Judi Julin , R.N. Nannybroker Inc.
25620 S.E. 15th St., Issaquah, WA 98027
206-624-1213
Fee 1st month salary of nanny

K.& D. Domestic Agency
7710 Balboa Ave, San Diego, CA 92123
619-296-0432
Fee one month salary of nanny

Kid Kare Agency
P.O. 7605, Shrewsbury, NJ 07702
908-747-2297
Fee 3 weeks of nanny's salary

KR&4 Kids Inc.
P.O. Box 1434, Madison, WI 53701
608-251-5324
Registration $40 Fee $900

Appendix B: Listing of nanny agencies and other services in the US.

Lousann Nanny Service
P.O.Box 310, Cheney, WA 99004-0310
509-534-9052

Love-n-care, Inc.
16 Bayberry Rd., Trenton, NJ 08618
800-538-1903
Registration $75 Fee $1,200

Maid In America
30 N. Raymond Ave., No. 406, Pasadena, CA 91103
818-792-9958

Mailibu Mamas Agency
22525 Pacific Coast Hwy ,Suite 203, Malibu, CA 90265
310-456-8113
Fee 10 % of the nanny's annual salary

Me and My Nannie & Senior Companions, Inc
1660 Akron Peninsula Rd, suite 104, Akron ,OH 44313
216-929-7040
Registration $250 Fee $1,000

Mommyworks ,Inc.
24331 Muirlands blvd. ,No.E, Lake Forest , CA 92630
714-830-9997
Registration $50 Fee $700

Moms Away
1015 Keith Ave., Berkley, CA 94708
510-559-9395
Fee one month of nanny's salary

Mother and Unborn Baby Care
Fort Worth ,TX 76116
817-870-2229

Mother's Aide, Inc.
P.O. Box 7088, Fairfax Station, VA 22039
703-250-0757
Registration $50 Fee $1,100

Mother's Care Referral Service, Inc
313 S. Ketch Dr., FT. Lauderdale, FL 33326
305-384-7141
Registration $50 Fee $250

Mother's Helper Agency
9454 Wilshire Blvd., No 600, Beverly Hills, CA 90212
310-271-1159, 1-800-942-2278
Registration $50 Fee $1,000

Mother's Helpmates
813 East Bloomingdale Ave Suite No. 160, Brandon, FL 33511
813-681-5183
Registration $150 Fee $450 to $650

Appendix B: Listing of nanny agencies and other services in the US.

Mother's- In- Deed
425 Sherman Ave ,Suit 130, Palo Alto, CA 94306
415-326-8570

Mother's and Newborn Homecare
123 Bellevue Ave, Newprot, RI 02840
401-849-2459

Mother's and Newborn Homecare
249 Wickenden St, Providence, RI 02903
401-751-2229

Nanny and Me
486 Little Turtle Lane, Cincinnati, OH 45244
513-528-8630
Registration $150 Fee $450

Nanny's Sitters Inc.
252 Ewing CT NW, Fort Walton, FL 32548
904-862-9652

Nannies Sitters Inc.
2200 W Highs Rd, Schaumburg, IL 60195
708-885-1700

Nannies Source Inc.
Wilton, CT 06897
203-762-9004

Nannies For Hire Inc.

430 SW 169 th Ter, Fort Lauderdale, FL 33326

305-932-5335

Namely Nannies

74 Greenwich Ave, Greenwich, CT 06830

203-629-8775

Fee $1,000

Nannie Source ,Inc.

P.O.Box 7371, Wilton, CT 06897

203-762-9004, 800-322-6264

Fee $1,000

Nannies by Daphane

P.O. Box 4505, Ithaca, NY 14850

607-277-Nani

Registration .$50 Fee $850

Nannies by Nita

6605 Clayton Ave. Suite 205, St.Louis, MO 63139

314-647-4717

Fee $800 to $1,000

Nannies Care

2701 Adrian St., San Diego, CA 92110

619-222-2490

Registration $250 Fee $900

Appendix B: Listing of nanny agencies and other services in the US.

Nannies For You
7624 Cantrell, Little Rock ,AR 72207
501-228-6264

Nannies Form E.S.P. Inc. Employment Search Professionals
533N. Hwy. 29, Newnan, GA 30263
404-253 9354
Registration .$75 Fee 9 % of the nanny's annual salary

Nannies From the Heartland
5490 Balsam Ln, Minneapolis, MN 55442
612-550-0219
Registration $100 Fee $750 to $850

Nannies Inc.
2903 Millwood Ave, Columbia, SC 29205
803-254-9264, 800-728-7643
Registration $200 Fee $500

Nannies Limited
1250 Kay Lane, Oakley, CA 94561
510-625-8382
Fee one month of nanny salary

Nannies Nook Inc.
3 Wanders Dr., Hingham, MA 02043
617 -749-8097, 800-542-4397
Registration $75 Fee $950 to $1350

Nannies of DuPage Inc.
P.O.Box 2368, Darien, IL 60559
708-963-6311
Fee $950

Nannies of Indiana
Washington St., Indianapolis, IN
317-897-6767
Registration $50

Nannies of Nebraska ,Inc.
125 S. 4th St. The Mcmill Bldg., Norfolk, NE 68701
402-379-2444, 402 379-4121
Registration $75 Fee $1,100

Nannies Plus
615 West Mt. Plesant Ave., Livingston, NJ 07039
201-992-5800, 800-752-0078
Registration $25 Fee $1,500

Nannies Preferred
1313 2nd West Hill Dr., Great Falls ,MT 59404
406-727-9897
Registration $50 Fee $495

Appendix B: Listing of nanny agencies and other services in the US.

Nannies Unlimited Agency
321 S. Beverly Dr. No 204, Beverly Hills, CA 90212
213-551-1621
Fee one month of nanny salary

Nannies USA East ,Inc.
28 Hereford Dr., Prince Junction, NJ 08550
609-799-4556
Registration $50 Fee $1,300

Nannies Who Care ,Inc.
1436 Dinnerbell Ln. E., Dunedin ,FL 34698
813-736-4295
Registration $75 Fee $725- $625-$425

Nannies with Dreams
RR1 , Box 9, Claremont, SD 57432
605-294-5896
Registration $100

Nanny Care Inc.
6315 Presidential Ct., Suite D, FT. Myers, FL 33919
813-433-1909, 800-728-2236
Registration $150

Nanny Concern Inc.
15 Mountain Rd., Wilton, CT 06897
203-544-9462
Fee $1,400

Nanny Connection
8331-202 Hempshire Place, Raleigh, NC 27613
919-870-1662
Registration $100 Fee 10 % of nanny's annual salary

Nanny Dimensions, Inc.
10560 Main St., Suite 513, Fairfax, VA 22030
703-691-0334
Registration $50 Fee is $1275

Nanny Finders, Inc.
110 Fairview Ave., Suite 201, Verona, NJ 07044
201-857-1700
Registration $100 Fee is $1085

Nanny Network, Inc.,
The 20145 N.E. 25th Avenue, Miami, FL 33180
305-932-5335
Registration $150 Fee is $1250

Appendix B: Listing of nanny agencies and other services in the US.

Nanny of America
4190 Telegraph, Suite 3300, Bloomfield Hills, MI 48302
313-540-4960
Fee varies.

Nanny Placement Agency
P.O. Box 1685, Reno, NV 89505
702-324-6561
Registration $75 Fee $925; $425

Nanny Poppins, Ltd.
301 Maple Avenue West Suite DE, Vienna, VA 22180
703-938-0444
Fee $975

Nanny Professionals, Inc.
P.O. Box 1253, Katy, TX 77492
713-392-4567
Registration $100, and 7% of nanny's annual salary

Nanny's & Granny's
6440 W. Coley, Las Vegas, NV 89102
702-364-5901
Registration $250 Fee $750

Nanny Search
52130 South Lakeshore Dr., Granger, IN 46530
219-277-8090
Registration temporary $35 Permanent $75 Fee $500

Nanny & Sitters, Inc.
2200 W. Higgins Road, Suite 105, Hoffman Estates, IL 60195
708-885-1700
Registration Live-in $1000 Out $750

National Nanny Network
6065 Roswell Rd., Suite 632, Atlanta, GA 30328
404-262-2585

Neighborhood Nannies, Inc.
205 Haddon Ave., Haddonfield, NJ 08033
609-795-5833
Registration $125 Fee 20% of nanny's annual salary

New World Nannies, Inc.
8706 Melwood Lane, Richmond, VA 23229
804-282-6128
Registration $50 Fee $400

Newport Nanny Placement Agency
18582 Beach Blvd., Suite 222, Huntington Beach, CA 92648
714-968-0380

Appendix B: Listing of nanny agencies and other services in the US.

North County Nannies
P.O. Box 460339, Escondido, CA 92046
619-480-0500
$1000 minimum live-in, $500 minimum live-out

Notre Maison, Inc.
6416 Carmel Rd., Suite 205, Charlotte, NC 28226
704-543-6240, 800-423-7895
Registration $100

Nurture Care,
Inc. 669 Airport Freeway, Suite 303, Hurst, TX 76053
817-285-8001
Registration $150- $300, live-in $1200, out $800

Nurturing Nannies
P.O. box 30576, Knoxville, TN 37930
615-691-2804

Oregon Nannies, Inc.
P.O. box 5551, Eugene, OR 97405
503-343-3755
Fee $1400

Original Nanny Service,
The 172 Institute Rd., Worcester, MA 01602
508-755-9284
Registration $75 Fee $1100

Overseas Custom Maid Nanny Line, Inc.
P.O. Box 249, East Norwich, NY 11732
516-624-9191

Parents Partners Line Inc.
2 Appletree Square, Suite 134, Bloomington, MN 55425
612-854-8594
Registration $100 Fee $800

Parent's Choice
100 Mill Plain Rd., Danbury, CT 06811
203-791-3891
Registration $100 Fee $800.

Patty's School Placements, Inc.
5213 Winchester Ln., Minneapolis, MN 55429
612-533-5219
Registration $100 Fee $850

Peace of Mind Nanny and Placement Services
509 Olive St. Suite 1200, St. Louis , MO 63101
314-241-2273
Registration $75 Fee $700

Philadelphia Nanny Network Inc.
The 145 West 67th Street ,No 31, New York, NY 10023
212-496-1213
Registration $50 Fee $1,500

Appendix B: Listing of nanny agencies and other services in the US.

Play Pals Child Services ,Inc.
HCR. 7 Box 124, Branson, MO 65616
417-336-2233

Poppin's Agency for Nannies
P.O. Box 361025, Grosse Pointe, MI 48236
313-884-9118

Potomac Nannies, Ltd.
7315 Wisconsin Ave Suite 331, West Bethseda, MD 20814
301-986-0048
Registration $75 Fee $700

Preferred Nannies Inc.
646-4 Main St., Port Jefferson ,NY 11777
516-474-4747, 800-323-1978
Fee $1,100

Prestige Nanny Service
P.O. Box 921538, Slylmar, CA 91392
818-364-6144
$25 Fee Not Specified.

Professional National Institute, Inc.
501 Fifth Ave. Suite 908, New York, NY 10017
212-692-9510
Registration $50 Fee 10 % of the nanny 's salary

Professional Nanny of Dallas
12810 Hillcrest, Suite 112, Dallas, TX 75230
214-661-1296
Registration $50 Fee 10 % of the nanny salary

Quality Care Associates ,Inc.
51 Purchase St., Rye, NY 10580
914-967-8254
Fee 3 times the nanny's salary

R & R Domestic Agency
280 Sylvan, Glencoe, IL 60022
708-835-2525
Fee one week of nanny's salary

Rent A Mom Of Colorado, Inc.
360 S. Monroe Suite 310, Denver, CO 80209
303-322-1399
Registration $,75 Placement $600 to $800

Rent A Parent Personnel Services
98 Main St., Suite 504, Triburon, CA 94920
415-435-2642
Fee one month of nanny's salary

Appendix B: Listing of nanny agencies and other services in the US.

Robin Kellner Agency
221 W. 57th St., New York, NY 10019
212-247-4141
Fee $1,350

Rose's Domestic Agency
6105 W. 6th St., Los Angeles, CA 90048
213-937-3196
Fee 1st month salary of the nanny

SilverSpoon Nanny Service
1601 S Van Buren, Enid , OK 73703
405-548-1099
Registration $100 Fee $1,200

Smiling Faces Inc.
1904 Byrd Ave Suite 309, Richmond, VA 23230
Registration $60 Fee $650 $450

Starkey and Associates ,Inc.
1410 High St., Denver, CO 80218
303-394-4908
Fee varies

Sterling Nannies, Inc.
10008 Rogart Rd., Silver Spring ,MD 20901
301-593-0069
Registration $50 Fee $1,000

Templeton Nannies ,Inc.
6300 Main St. Suite 403, Kansas, MO 64113
816-444-1888
Registration $95, Fee $950

Tender Care Nannies Placement Agency
19022 Wisconsin Drive, Chippewa Falls, WI 54729
715-723-7050
Registration $50 Fee $800

TGIF Peopleworks
P.O. Box 828, Old Lyme, CT 06371
203-434-2526

The Connection School for Nannies
232 Skitchwaug Trail, Springfield, VT 05156
802-885-3556
Registration $100 Fee varies

The Executive Nanny
1428 Daryll Lane, Roanoke, TX 76262
817-23-nanny
Registration $100 Fee 10 % of nanny's salary

The Governess Agency
4655 Cass No. 405 R, San Diego, CA 92109
619-270-8311
Fee one month's of nanny's salary

Appendix B: Listing of nanny agencies and other services in the US.

The Governess Agency
125 E Baker St Costa, Mesa, CA 92626
714-979-6200

The Governess Agency
3111 Camino Del Rio N, San Diego, CA 92108
619-528-2244

Templeton Nannies
Kanas City, MO 64114
816-444-1888

The Minute Women
Concord, MA 01742
508-369-3171

The Minute Women
111 Union Whar No.-A, Boston, MA 02109
617-227-1889

The Minute Women
49 Waltham St, Lexington, MA 02173
617-862-3300

The Mom Connection
6060 Sunrise Vista Dr., Citrus Heights, CA
916-722-5008
Fee $775 to $825

The Nanny Connection
10628 Looking Glass Rd., Richmond, VA 23235
804-379-9314
Registration $65 Placement fee $490- $750

The Nanny Corporation
325 E. Eisenhower Parkway, Suite 106, Ann Arbor, MI 48108
313-769-5265, 313-258-6330
Registration $150 Fee $975-1075

The Nanny Search
Granger, IN 46530
219-277-8090

The Nanny Solution, Inc.
P.O. Box 10278, Bedford, NH 03110
603-472-2719, 603-472-8494
Registration $95, Fee $295- $695

The Nanny Source, Inc.
415 Route 10, Randolph, NJ 07869
201-328-1619

T.L..C., Inc.
5424- 10 Sunol Blvd., Suite 111, Pleanton, CA 94566
510-426-8028
Fee one month of nanny's salary

Appendix B: Listing of nanny agencies and other services in the US.

TLC For Kids ,Inc.
7301 Tulane, St. Louis, MO 63130
314-752-5660
Registration $50 Fee $400 to $850

TLC For Kids, Inc.
P. O. Box 50637, Nashville, TN 37205
615-385- 297-1914
Registration $50 Fee $750

TLC Sitters of Atlanta, Inc.
1262 Concord Rd., Smyrna, GA 30080
404-435-6250
Registration $150 Fee varies

TLC Unlimited ,Inc.
341-11 College Rd. Suite 141, Wilmington, NC 28403
919-799-5132
Registration $100 Fee $100 to 5 % of nanny's salary

Town and Country Nannies ,Inc.
2384 South Broadway, Denver, CO 80210
305-744-6112
Registration $150 Fee Varies

Appendix B: Listing of nanny agencies and other services in the US.

Umbrella Child Care Services
3508 W 22nd St., Minneapolis, MN 55416
612-929-0877
Registration $60 to $180 Fee $300 to $900

Victorias Nannies,
Inc. 7721 5 Miles Rd., Cincinnati, OH 45230
513-232-0441
Registration $250 Fee $750

White House Nannies ,Inc.
4733 Bethesda Ave., Suite 804, Bethesda, MD 20814
301-654-5506

Yankee Sitters P.O.
Box 475, Webster, MA 01570
508-949-6244
Registration $75 Fee $800

Additonal books are available through Mother's Heplmates Publications.

Mother's Helpmates
813 E. Bloomingdale Ave. #160
Brandon, FL 33511
(813) 681-5183
(800) 221-5183

Mother's Helpmate Guide to Child Care, Nannies and Companions

Book Order Form

Name____

Addres______________________________________

City__________________________ State______ Zip____________

Phone_______________________________________

Price includes shipping and handling. Florida residents include sale tax of 6.5%.

			Total
Cost	$ 19.95 each	# of Books_____	___________
Florida Sales Tax 6.5%			___________
		Total	___________
